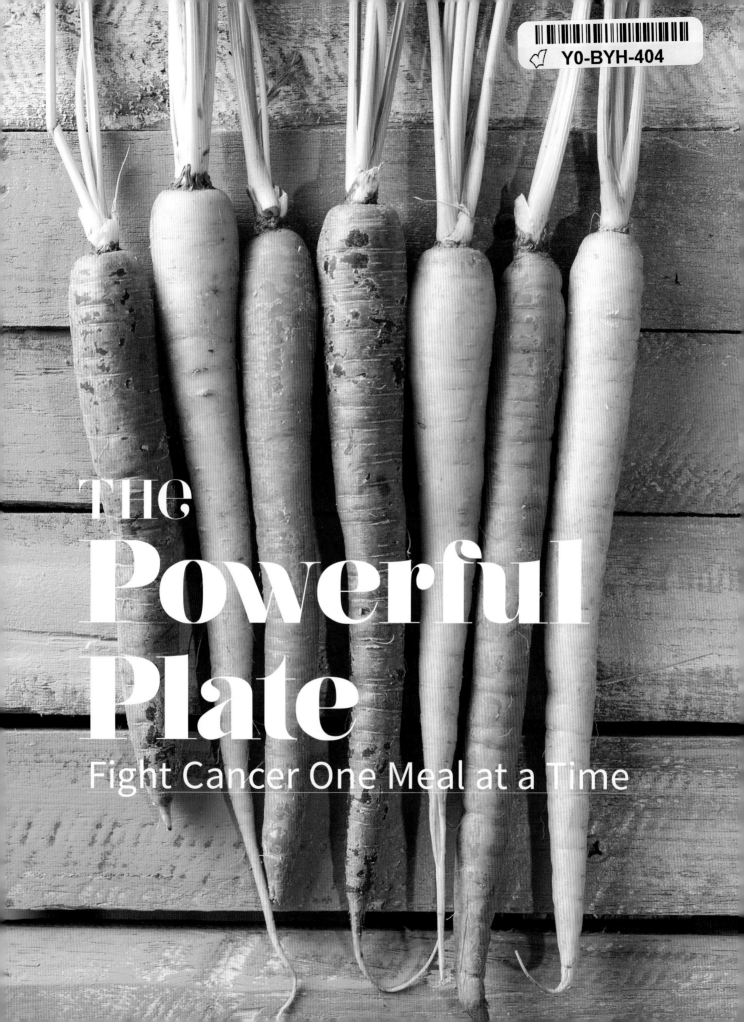

The
Powerful
Plate

Fight Cancer One Meal at a Time

Graphic design provided by Lifestyle Canada Education Service

Library of Congress Cataloging-in-Publication Data

Names: Donkor, Afia, author.
Title: The powerful plate : fight cancer one meal at a time / Afia Donkor.
Description: Nampa : Pacific Press Publishing Association, 2019. | Includes bibliographical references. |
    Summary: "A study of the foods that fight cancer and how this influences our spiritual health"—
    Provided by publisher.
Identifiers: LCCN 2019030540 | ISBN 9780816366026 (paperback) | ISBN 9780816366033 (kindle edition)
Subjects: LCSH: Cancer—Diet therapy. | Cancer—Nutritional aspects.
Classification: LCC RC271.D52 D66 2019 | DDC 616.99/40654—dc23
LC record available at https://lccn.loc.gov/2019030540

October 2019

DISCLAIMER:

Dedication

Very rarely is a book dedicated to its author.
The Powerful Plate *is an exception.*
Afia Donkor spent countless hours in researching and designing
this book. The project would never have been accomplished
without her dedication, faith, and sacrificial giving.

Afia suddenly passed away from health complications
on November 11, 2017.

At iHeal, we have already seen many lives changed as a result
of her work. We hope that you, too, can find healing through the
legacy you hold in your hands.

—The iHeal Team

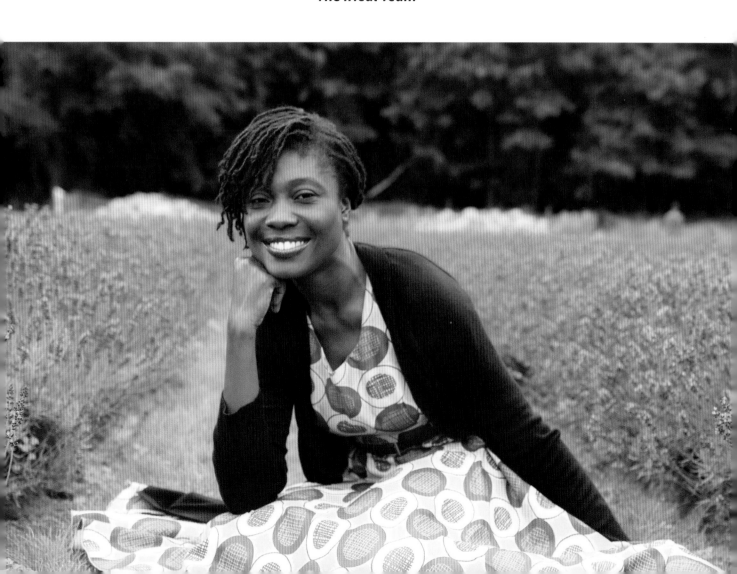

Contents

Let Food Be Your Medicine

Norman's Miracle 8

The "C" Word 10

Cancer: What Is It? 10

Lifestyle, Food, and Cancer 13

Foods That Help

Fruits 17

Berries 19

Apples 20

Tomatoes 23

Grapes 24

Pomegranates 25

Dried Fruits 26

All Fruits 27

Vegetables 29

Carrots 31

Beta-Carotene Rich Vegetables 32

Cruciferous Vegetables 35

The Allium Family 36

All Vegetables 37

Whole Grains 39

Whole Grains 40

Legumes 43

Legumes 45

Healthy Fats 49

Nuts 50

Flaxseeds 51

Olives and Olive Oil 52

Avocados 53

Foods That Hurt

Animal Products 57

Animal Protein 58

Dairy and Animal Fat 60

A Reason to Hope 63

Alcohol 65

Alcohol 66

Sugar, Salt, and Spices 69

Sugar 71

Salt 72

Spicy Foods 73

Recipes

Breakfast 77

Pumpkin French Toast 79

Steel-Cut Oats 81

Berry Waffles..83

Granola...85

Nut Milk...87

Multigrain Flax Bread...89

Very Berry Smoothie...91

Tofu Veggie Scramble...93

Mains..95

Black Bean Burgers...97

Spinach-Basil Pesto..99

Lentil Stew...101

Black-Eyed Bean Stew...103

Tofu Salad..105

Vegan Mac and Cheese..107

Broccoli "Cheese" Potatoes...109

Sweet Potato Burritos..111

Creamy Rice 'n' Sprouts...113

Hummus...115

Tomato Soup..117

Veggie Wrap With "Cream Cheese"...119

Salads...121

Cilantro Citrus Slaw..123

Romaine Salad With Creamy Walnut Dressing...........................125

Broccoli Salad..127

Sweet Treats..129

Baked Peaches..131

Oatmeal-Walnut Cookies..133

Banana Ice Cream..135

Crispy Sunflower Bars...137

Grape-Pomegranate Sorbet...139

Carrot Cake..141

Fruit Parfait...143

Beyond the Plate

It Begins With Eight...147

Nutrition..149

Exercise..153

Water..154

Sunlight..156

Temperance...157

Air...158

Rest...161

Trust...162

Your Turn...165

Step 1: How Healthy Is Your Lifestyle?.......................................166

Step 2: Personal Goals...167

Step 3: My Commitment...167

Endnotes...168

Let Food Be Your Medicine

The concept that Western diseases are lifestyle-related and therefore potentially preventable and reversible is the most important medical discovery of the twentieth century.

—Denis Burkitt, MD

Norman's Miracle

On a Tuesday afternoon in October, I was bustling around my apartment getting ready for work when I received a text notification. I glanced down at the screen and read: "*Afia…the specialist told me I have lymphoma cells in my throat.*" The story of that text, of its sender, and of what happened next is a powerful, living example of why the message of this book is important. But the story begins in an unlikely place—a law office six years earlier.

I was a brand-new employee working in a small law office in southern Ontario. On my first day my boss handed me a large box filled from top to bottom with files and told me to have at it. That was my introduction to the practice of law in Canada, and when I was called to the bar in Ontario a year later, my work responsibilities expanded.

As part of those responsibilities, I began working from time to time with a client named Norman. As I got to know him, we would often talk about a number of things, including faith and health. But as the years passed and my responsibilities and role in the office changed, I saw Norman less and less until I lost sight of him entirely. It was with immense shock, then, that years later I saw Norman, wide-eyed and haggard, making his slow and painful way toward the front door of our office.

Little by little I learned, first from others, then from Norman himself, of the serious health challenges he had been facing. Then one morning, Norman said something to me that took me completely by surprise. "Afia, I want you to help me."

I sat down with Norman early one morning with a pen and a questionnaire. Aside from my work as a lawyer I had volunteered for a few years with a charity that, among other things, made it a mission to teach Canadians the principles of healthy living. The charity had created a questionnaire that sought to bring out, in detail, the state of a person's health habits. So for nearly two hours I went through the questions with Norman. As we talked, a terrible picture of his health challenges emerged. He suffered from extreme anxiety; depression; confusion; multiple strokes; high blood pressure; sciatica; elevated PSA levels; severe; crippling back pain; throat constriction; and chronic, severe insomnia. I was almost breathless with the scope of problems and wondered how one body could contain them all.

But as I turned to the section of the questionnaire that dealt with lifestyle practices, I uncovered many things that concerned me. Norman drank very little water, ate out frequently, ate very few fruits and vegetables, consumed high amounts of dairy, and in general knew very little about how to take care of his health. But he was eager to learn.

I went home with the checklist and sat down to think. Then I made a decision. Calling Norman, I said, "Norman, I'm going to cook for you."

Hippocrates once declared, "Let food be thy medicine and medicine be thy food." I believe that this statement reveals an important truth about a daily aspect of our lives. In the face of Norman's challenges, I felt a desire to put that statement to a real-life test. Norman was willing, so we made plans and stepped forward to see where this journey would take us.

We began with a modified fast. For several days, Norman drank fresh vegetable juice three times a day. On the first day of the fast, he fell asleep for several hours during the day. The second day, he fell asleep before 10:00 P.M., something unheard of for him, and slept through the night. By the third day, Norman was calling the juice "magic juice." The swelling in his body, especially his legs, had disappeared. He said his body felt light like a cloud, and he could think more clearly and concentrate better. Even the pain in his sciatic nerve had lessened.

When the fast ended, we moved on to phase two. I prepared and packaged various plant-based foods, including steel-cut oats with cashew milk, homemade multigrain flax bread, soups filled with beans and vegetables, homemade soy milk, and homemade granola. I prepared a menu and labeled the containers so things could be as easy for Norman as possible. All he needed to do was warm up the food and add fresh fruits and vegetables.

Before our eyes, we began to see a transformation. Norman lost weight steadily and reported with amazement that while he now ate less, he felt full for much longer periods of time. His blood pressure dropped and other medical markers began to improve. Even better, he loved the food he was eating and his former cravings for meat and other animal products completely disappeared.

One of the things Norman had especially suffered from was severe, overwhelming back pain. Persistent and even extreme medical interventions hadn't helped, and he had come to the place where he was considering physician-assisted suicide to end his suffering. But five days into the fast I learned that another acquaintance of mine, Norwill, had suffered from similar problems and had found an unconventional solution—an herb called comfrey.

I had always been suspicious about such claims, but I called Norwill and he told me his story. Then I began to do research myself. I found a study posted on the website for the National Institutes of Health in the United States that affirmed comfrey's effectiveness in reducing back pain.[1] I figured it couldn't hurt to try, and it might even help. So after getting Norman's consent, Norwill made a comfrey oil preparation for him and helped him apply it topically nearly every evening. In three weeks, Norman's pain was gone. His unsteady movements, his sudden falls, his suffering, all were gone. In three weeks, he was a new, healthy, lively person.

It was October, two months into the start of our experiment, that I received the text from Norman saying he had lymphoma. Norman explained that earlier that year, his doctors had done some tests and discovered the disease, but for whatever reason, the results had been overlooked and he was never told.

Now the doctors, fearing the cancer had spread all over his body, urgently scheduled further testing and treatment.

Norman was extremely worried. He had every right to be. But I reminded him that he had, for two months, been on a very different path. He had been making better dietary choices and he felt better. Maybe, just maybe, things had improved.

Norman went in for testing and then we waited for the results. Two weeks later, he sent me the following:

"Hi Afia, I know you could be busy but can't wait to tell you. My lungs, my abdominals, and my bladder are completely clear. They only found swelling in my lower throat/esophagus. They don't know where the lymphoma cells went. They canceled my chemotherapy treatment for now to do further tests to find out where the lymphoma cells found by the biopsy went. Praise God. Praise God. Praise God. I got new life."[2]

Norman's story, while remarkable, is not isolated. There is something about good food that makes a tangible impact on health. It is true that not everyone will experience the dramatic and rapid changes Norman experienced. It is also true that dietary changes alone are not always enough. Traditional medicine plays an important role in supporting the health of a community. Still, the fact remains that Hippocrates was right. Good food, combined with other healthy lifestyle choices, can be like medicine to the body. It can help the body achieve and maintain good health—one seed, one nut, one grain at a time. This book seeks to help you understand why.

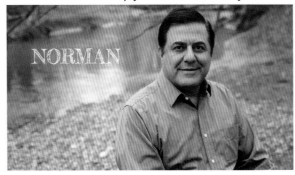

The "C" Word

Two in five Canadians will develop it in their lives, and one in four will lose their lives because of it.[3] In the United States, one in two men and one in three women are at risk of developing it, while 22 percent of men and 19 percent of women will die from it.[4] The numbers are startling. Behind them is the reality of a disease so devastating and so widespread that it has become the focus of national and international attention. That disease is cancer.

For many, cancer is a deeply personal reality. Some have suffered or are suffering from it, and others have a neighbor, a friend, or a loved one whose life has been changed because of it. The suffering and loss that this disease has brought throughout the world is incalculable. It strikes in all directions, claiming the lives of children, adults, the rich, and the poor in every part of the world.

Cancer can sometimes seem hard to understand, predict, and prevent. Because of this, many feel helpless against it, wondering if they, or their loved ones, will be the next to fall under its shadow. But as scientists are gaining understanding about how our bodies work, the veil that seems to enshroud cancer is being lifted, revealing hope for those who choose to grasp it.

This book seeks to shine a light on a simple truth: cancer is not inevitable. The secret to greatly reducing your risk lies in one little word—*choice*. An ounce of prevention is worth pounds and pounds of cure. Whether you are currently suffering from the disease or seeking to prevent it, simple, healthy lifestyle changes matter. They help increase your odds of avoiding, and even overcoming, cancer.

Cancer: What Is It?

Cancer is a term used to describe abnormal cell behavior. Ordinarily, all of our cells follow set orders and procedures. They grow at certain times, perform certain functions, divide at certain times, and die at certain times. But sometimes the DNA in our cells gets damaged, and this damage derails the normal, ordered functions of our cells.

Carcinogenesis is the process by which normal cells are transformed into cancerous cells. It takes place in three basic stages: initiation, promotion, and progression.[5]

- **Initiation** happens when a carcinogen (a substance with the potential to cause cancer) alters the DNA of a cell, causing a mutation.
- **Promotion** happens when compounds called promoters help mutated cells reproduce at rapid, abnormal rates, forming tumors. If the abnormal growth remains in just one part of the body, the tumor is benign.
- **Progression** is when mutated cells grow uncontrollably and take on aggressive characteristics. When a tumor begins to invade neighboring tissue, it is cancerous. When a tumor begins to spread to other parts of the body, it is said to metastasize.

"

This book seeks to shine a light on a simple truth: cancer is not inevitable. The secret to greatly reducing your risk lies in one little word—choice.

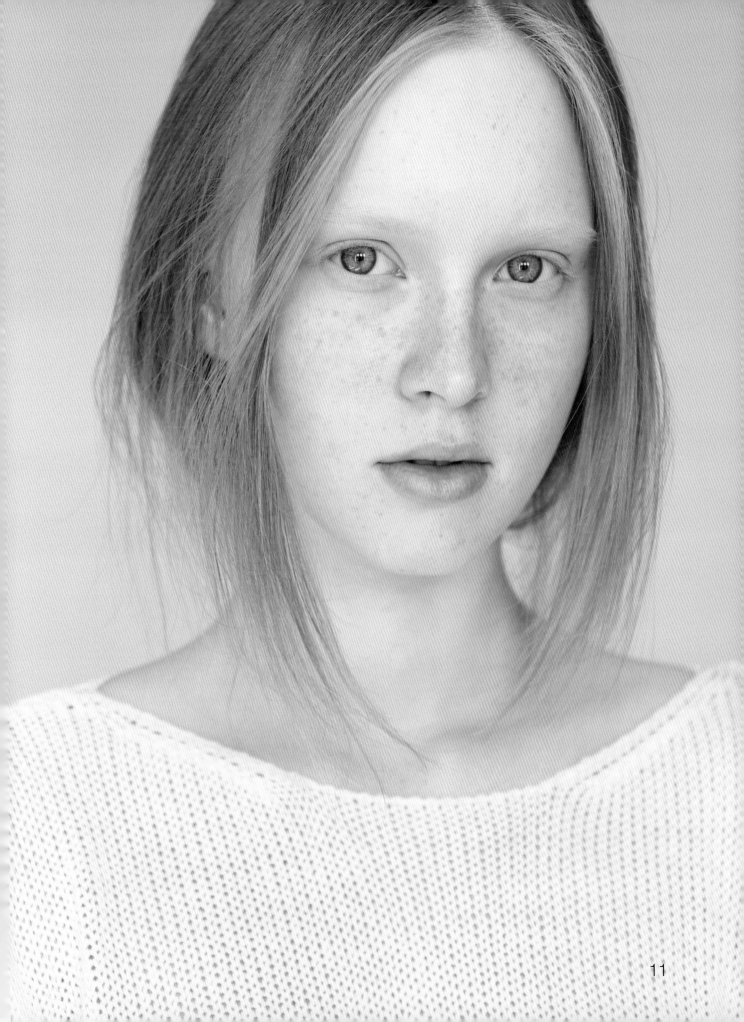

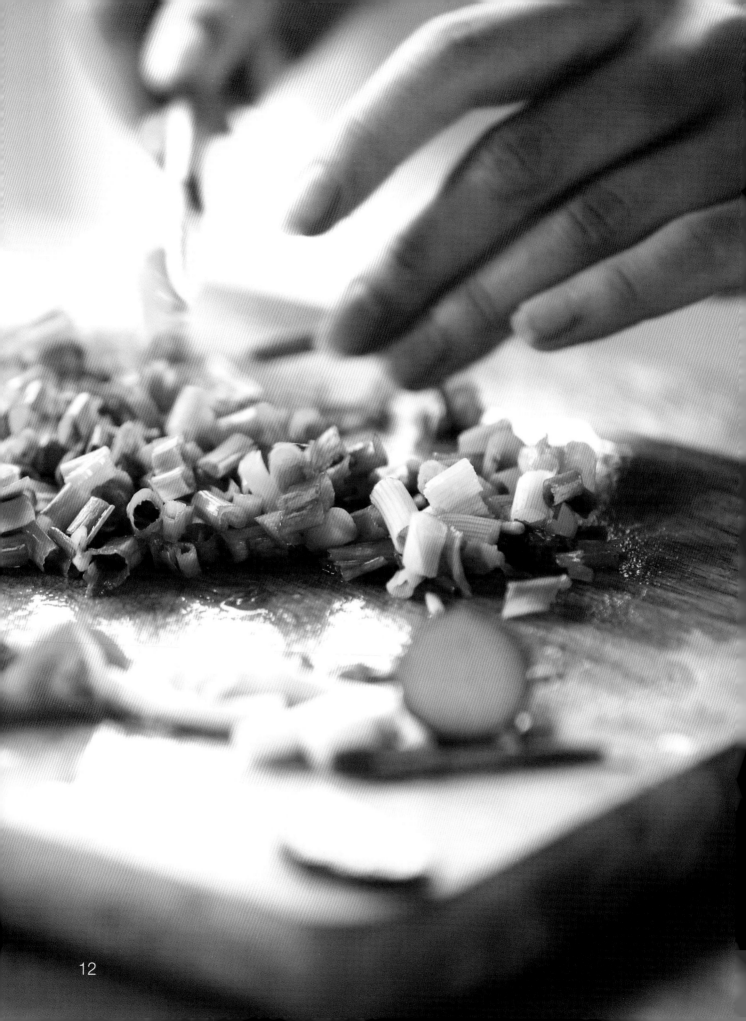

Lifestyle, Food, and Cancer

Many studies have established a link between certain lifestyle behaviors and cancer risk. These studies reveal a simple yet profound truth—cancer is preventable. Worldwide, only 5–10 percent of cancer cases are caused by genetic defects. The remaining 90–95 percent come as a result of lifestyle choices and some environmental factors:

- 30–35 percent of all cancer cases are linked to diet.

- 25–30 percent of all cancer cases are due to tobacco.

- 15–20 percent of all cancer cases are due to infections.

- The remaining cancer cases come from factors like stress, physical activity, environmental pollutants, and radiation.[6]

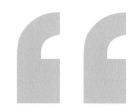

Over the years, consumers have heard warning after warning about the latest dangerous chemicals that cause cancer and threaten health and life. From nitrites to weed killers to chemical dough conditioners in bread, many products in the environment and in our foods have generated fear and alarm in the general public. While concerns about carcinogens and contaminants are understandable, the statistics just cited suggest that our focus may be misplaced. As scientists uncover more information about the link between diet and health, it is increasingly evident that the everyday foods we eat may have a greater impact on our health than the environmental polution and artificial chemicals we fear.

The fact is that individual choice is the single most important factor that determines whether a person will overcome, or be overcome by, cancer. That is *great* news. We choose what we eat, we choose what we drink, and we choose what we do. To a large degree, then, our health is in our own hands, and this should give us hope. Through our choices, we have a say in the kind of health we will have and we can strive to make it the very best health possible.

We spoke earlier about the three stages of carcinogenesis that transform normal cells into cancer cells. These again are initiation, promotion, and progression. The impact of lifestyle in cancer prevention plays a hugely important role because it touches on all three stages. This is especially true when it comes to diet. It is impossible to avoid contact with all carcinogens (the substances that initiate the cancer process). They are in the food we eat, the water we drink, and the air we breathe. But the lifestyle choices we make, from exercising to eating certain foods, will determine whether our bodies will be equipped to handle carcinogens or be overwhelmed by them.

This book seeks to help you understand the role food plays in carcinogenesis. We will explain just how our cells interact with the foods we give them. As we do this, we will better understand just how food helps our bodies or hurts them.

To a large degree . . . our health is in our own hands, and this should give us hope. Through our choices, we have a say in the kind of health we will have and we can strive to make it the very best health possible.

Foods That Help

Let food be thy medicine and
medicine be thy food.
—Hippocrates

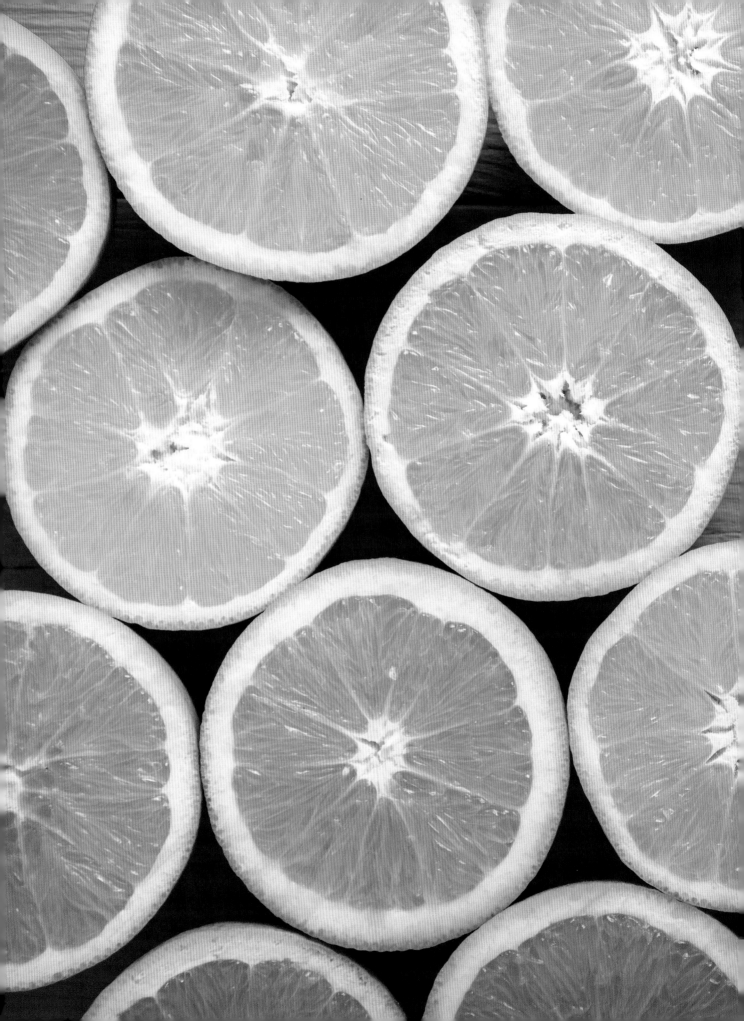

Fruits

Fruits are nature's sweet treat. They also come complete with some sweet nutritional benefits. They are full of antioxidants and phytochemicals that play a crucial role in maintaining health and lowering cancer risk. For example, one study found that those who eat fruit more than once a day have only a 25 percent chance of getting lung cancer, compared with those who eat fruit less than three times a week.[7] Many other studies have consistently found that eating fruit results in reduced cancer risk.

A number of fruits and fruit categories have received a lot of attention and have been praised for their cancer-fighting properties. We will review a few of these categories here. Remember, however, that scientists are only beginning to understand the nutritional impact of fruits of all varieties. All fruits hold the promise of improved health, even when it comes to cancer. So make a wide variety of fruits from a wide variety of categories an everyday part of life. If you do, you will reap positive results.

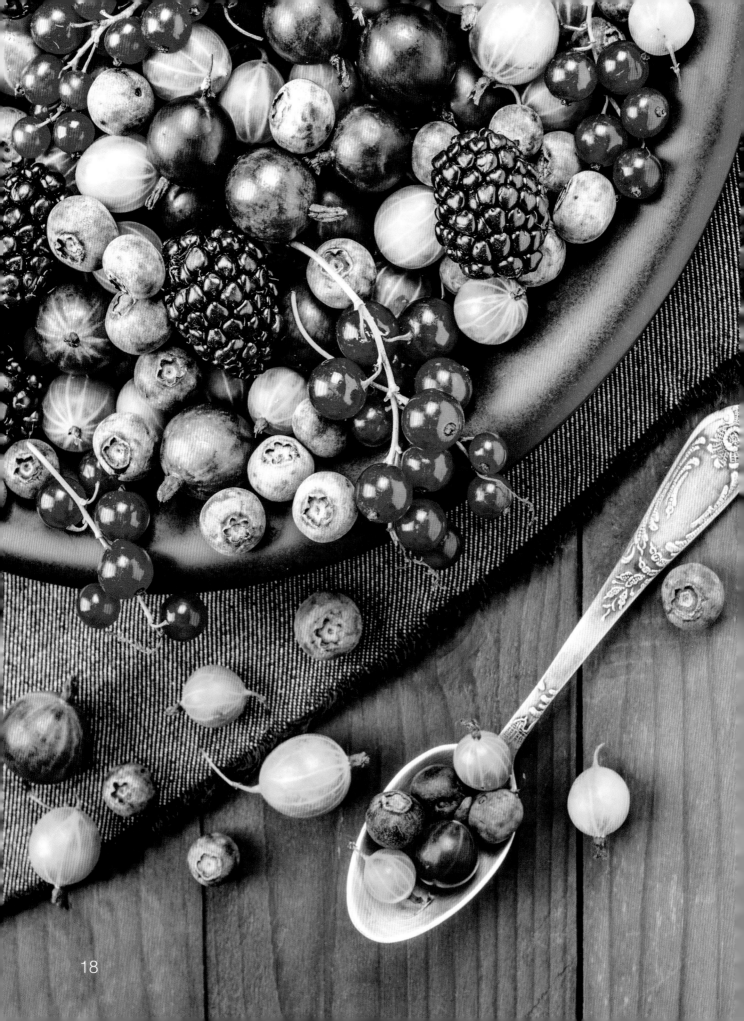

Berries

According to the American Institute for Cancer Research, "Berries may be among the most beneficial fruits to eat for cancer prevention."[8] Why? Because they contain a substance called antioxidants.

Antioxidants are molecules that help prevent and even fight cancer. This is because they help prevent oxidation. Oxidation is a chemical process that produces free radicals that damage cells and their DNA. This damage leads to cancerous mutations and causes cells to die.

Molecules like vitamins, minerals, and phytochemicals have powerful antioxidant properties. Together, these molecules protect against damage from oxidation. They also help repair damage that has already been done. Antioxidants in berries affect the growth of cancerous cells. They even help trigger the death of cancer cells, a process called apoptosis.[9] Berry antioxidants also make cancer cells more sensitive to chemotherapy. This makes them more responsive to treatment.[10]

But antioxidants are not the only name in the game. Berries also contain fiber. Fiber protects against cancer because it adds bulk to foods and helps move waste quickly out of the body. This is important because of the following facts:

- Added bulk in fiber-rich foods gives a sensation of fullness when eating. This helps to control the amount of food eaten which helps to prevent obesity, a significant cancer risk.
- Waste often contains carcinogens, so the more quickly and efficiently waste is removed from the body, the less our cells are exposed to carcinogens.[11]

Laboratory research on the protective effects of berries has made some promising findings. For instance, one study found that a diet of freeze-dried black raspberries or strawberries inhibits esophageal cancer in rats by 30–60 percent, and colon cancer by up to 80 percent.[12]

As with anything, when it comes to berries, variety is the spice of life. From blueberries to strawberries to the many varieties in between, each berry has its own unique antioxidant makeup and provides unique benefits. So mix things up and make a variety of berries a regular addition to your diet.

> "
>
> Antioxidants are molecules that help prevent and even fight cancer.

RECOMMENDATIONS:

- Eat at least one serving of berries (1 cup raw) 3–4 times per week, and try different varieties.
- Enjoy berries raw, as the antioxidant levels of berries are greatly reduced when cooked.
- If possible, go organic. A number of studies have found that organic berries have higher antioxidant levels than the nonorganic variety.
- Frozen berries are an excellent alternative to fresh. They are picked when ripe, which is the time when antioxidant levels are at their highest, and they are nutrient stable when frozen.

The old adage "an apple a day keeps the doctor away" may very well be true when it comes to preventing cancer. This is because the fiber and antioxidants in apples help fight the growth and spread of cancerous cells.

- Pectin, a dietary fiber in apples, acts as a scavenger to remove mutagens out of the body. Mutagens cause cell mutations that can lead to cancerous cells. Apple pectin also increases the mass of our stool and moves it quickly out of the colon. This dilutes the concentration of mutagens and eliminates them from the body before they do harm.[13]

- Apples contain an antioxidant molecule called quercetin. The highest concentration of quercetin is found in the apple peel. This antioxidant protects cells from free-radical damage and fights against the development of mutated, cancerous cells.[14]

- Apples have anti-inflammatory properties, particularly because of the antioxidant quercetin. This is important because chronic inflammation breeds the perfect conditions for the growth of cancer cells: it inhibits cell death, stimulates cell growth, and gives cells abundant sources of food in the form of new blood cells. All this provides the perfect environment for cancer growth. However, the chemicals in apples help prevent this from happening.[15]

From molecular science to real-world experience, apples are making a valuable impact on cancer prevention and treatment:

- People who eat one or more apples each day reduce their risk of developing colorectal cancer by 30 percent, breast cancer by 24 percent, and prostate cancer by 7 percent.[16]

- Those who consume the greatest amounts of apples, onions, and white grapefruits experience a 40–50 percent decrease in the risk of lung cancer.[17]

- Individuals who eat one apple or more a day decrease their risk of developing a number of cancers, including breast, prostate, and colorectal cancer.[18]

> Individuals who eat one apple or more a day decrease their risk of developing a number of cancers, including breast, prostate, and colorectal cancer.

RECOMMENDATIONS:

- Eat apples regularly. An apple a day may keep the oncologist away!
- Eat the whole apple, as the antioxidants in apples are concentrated in their skins. For instance, about 80 percent of quercetin is found in the apple peel.[19]
- Consider purchasing organic apples. Traditional apples are high on the list of pesticide-contaminated produce.[20]

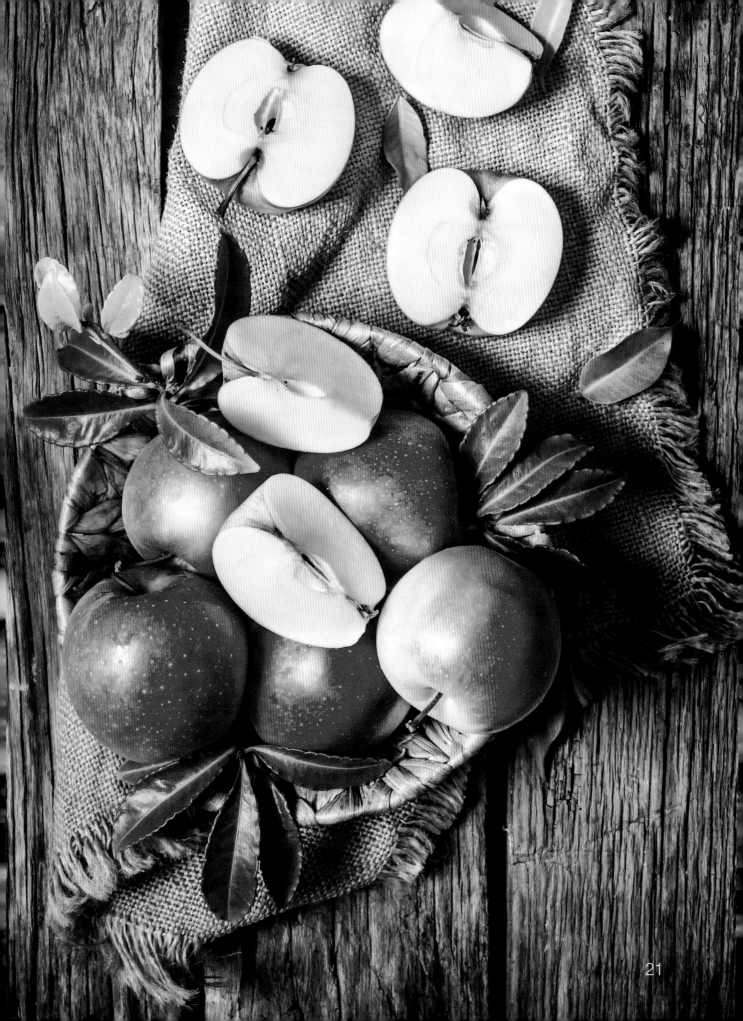

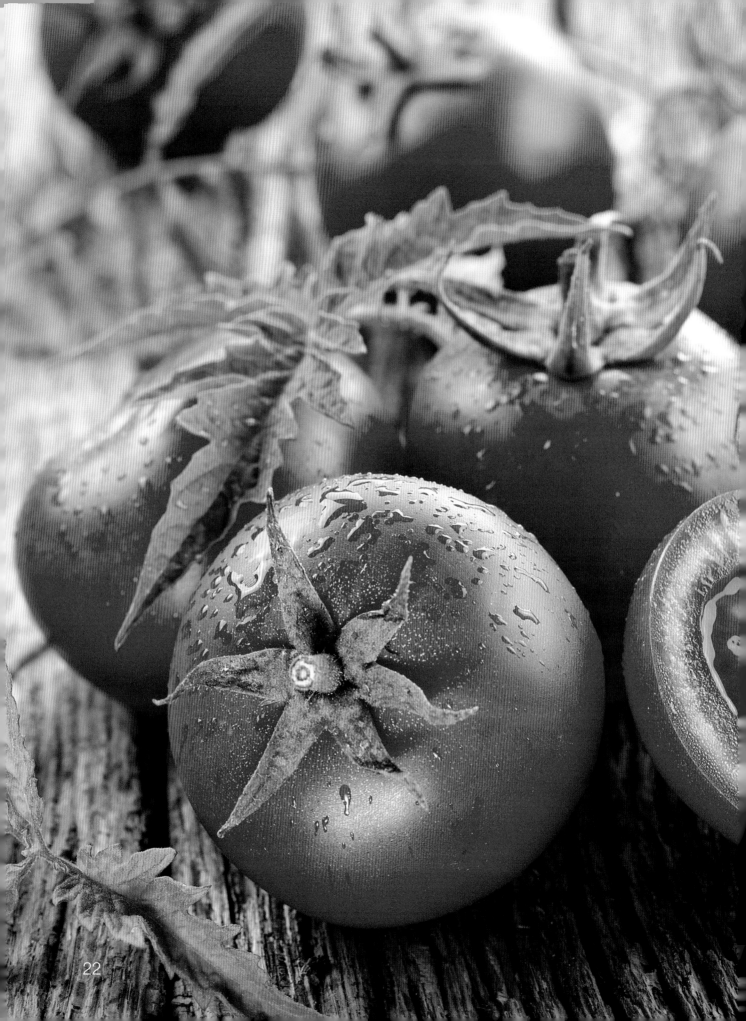

Tomatoes

Tomatoes are fruits with impressive cancer-fighting qualities. In fact, the tomato's bright pigment reveals its antioxidant capabilities.

Carotenoids are the molecules behind the red, orange, and yellow pigments in fruits and vegetables. The carotenoid lycopene, present in tomatoes, has drawn a lot of attention because of its antioxidant capabilities. Tomatoes are also rich in other antioxidants, including beta-carotene and vitamin C. When it comes to tomatoes, lycopene, and cancer, here is what the research is saying:

- Dietary intake of lycopene, provided mainly by tomatoes, results in a 31 percent reduction in pancreatic cancer risk.[21]

- Men who have the highest intake of lycopene lower their risk of developing prostate cancer by 21 percent. Men who eat the highest amounts of tomatoes and tomato products reduce their risk of prostate cancer by 35 percent, and of aggressive prostate cancer by 53 percent, compared with men who eat the lowest amounts.[22]

- Smokers who consume the highest amounts of fruits and vegetables, particularly carotenoids, tomatoes, and tomato-based products, reduce their risk of lung cancer. The consumption of lycopene-rich foods, for instance, reduces risk by 28 percent.[23]

- Unlike other fruits, when it comes to tomatoes, cooking is the way to go. This is because lycopene content *increases* when tomatoes are cooked. Also, lycopene is a fat-soluble molecule so the presence of fat improves our body's ability to absorb it.[24]

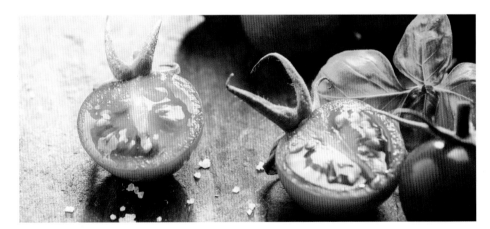

> Men who eat the highest amounts of tomatoes and tomato products reduce their risk of prostate cancer by 35 percent, and of aggressive prostate cancer by 53 percent, compared with men who eat the lowest amounts.

RECOMMENDATIONS:

- Regularly include tomatoes and tomato products in your diet.
- Cook tomatoes with a little fat to maximize lycopene content and absorption.
- Combine raw tomatoes with a little fat to increase lycopene absorption. For example, add chunks of avocado to a tomato salad, or drizzle a little olive oil on a salad with tomatoes.

Grapes

Grape compounds are often praised for their contributions to cardiovascular health. Something else that is being heard through the grapevine is that grapes may protect against cancer. Laboratory studies have discovered that certain compounds found in grapes protect against all three stages of cancer development (initiation, promotion, and progression). They have been shown to

- prevent the formation of cancerous cells
- arrest the progression of cancer cells and
- induce apoptosis (cell death) in cancer cells.[25]

It is not surprising that grapes seem to protect against, and to fight, the growth and rapid increase of cancer cells. This is because grapes have a number of benefits going for them. They are high in fiber and rich in antioxidants. One grape antioxidant that has received a lot of attention is resveratrol. Resveratrol has anti-inflammatory properties[26] and has also been shown to inhibit estrogenic activity. This is important because some cancers, such as breast cancer, are estrogen-dependent (see page 51 for more information on the link between estrogen and estrogen-dependent cancers).[27]

> Laboratory studies have discovered that certain compounds found in grapes protect against all three stages of cancer.

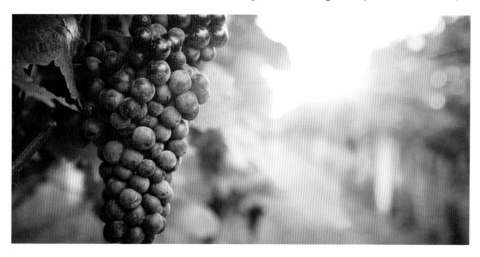

RECOMMENDATIONS:

- Eat a serving of grapes several times per week.
- Eat whole grapes. Their beneficial components are heavily concentrated in their skins and seeds.
- If available, buy grapes with seeds and consume their seeds. Sixty to seventy percent of grape polyphenols (molecules that one study referred to as "one of the most potent natural antioxidants") are found in the seeds.[28]
- All varieties of grapes are healthy, but consider choosing darker-hued varieties as they provide the greatest health benefit. Red, purple, and black grapes contain higher concentrations of resveratrol and other antioxidants.
- If possible, try to buy organic grapes as grapes are high on the list of pesticide-contaminated produce.[29]

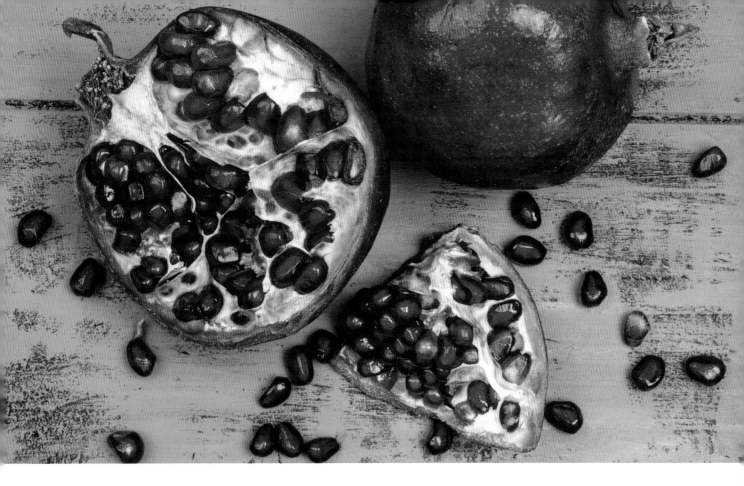

Pomegranates

You may have seen the POM Wonderful juice bottles in the grocery store and heard something about how pomegranates are good for the heart. Well, scientific research is now suggesting that pomegranates may also have a role in cancer prevention.

- Certain chemicals found in pomegranates inhibit estrogenic activity. This is promising for breast cancer research.[30]

- Men who drank an 8-ounce glass of pomegranate juice every day and received no other treatment had a 12 percent decrease in cancer cell proliferation and a 17 percent increase in cancer cell death.[31]

The promise of pomegranates in cancer prevention and treatment is perhaps not terribly surprising. This is because pomegranates are very high in antioxidants that protect and repair cells.

RECOMMENDATIONS:

- Enjoy fresh pomegranates as an addition to your fruit and vegetable intake.
- Add pomegranate juice as an occasional fruit juice treat.
- Pomegranate seeds freeze well, so take advantage of the moments when pomegranates are in season by buying them in bulk. Remove the seeds from the fruit and freeze them in freezer-safe containers. Then enjoy them sprinkled over cereals, in oatmeal, or all on their own for weeks and months at a time.

Dried Fruits

They are packed into tiny boxes, strewn through trail mix, and sprinkled on top of salads and oatmeal. But those small, wrinkled pieces of fruit are more than just a garnish or a sweet treat: they play a meaningful part in keeping us healthy, particularly when it comes to cancer.

- **Dried fruits are high in phenols.**[32] Phenols are antioxidants found only in plant foods. They have both antioxidant and anti-inflammatory effects on the body.[33] Their antioxidant capabilities protect against damage from free radicals (which can produce cancerous cells) and repair damaged cells. As anti-inflammatory molecules, they work to counteract inflammation in the body. This helps keep the body from creating environments conducive to cancer cell growth.

- **Dried fruits are high in fiber.**[34] This is important because fiber scavenges mutagens, traps cancerous cells, and moves them quickly out of our bodies before they can do lasting damage.

Studies show that those who regularly incorporate dried fruits in their diet reap tangible benefits:

- People who regularly eat dates, raisins, and other dried fruits reduce their risk of developing pancreatic cancer compared with those who rarely or never eat dried fruits.[35]

- Individuals who eat dried fruits between three and five times each week reduce their risk of developing prostate cancer by 40 percent.[36]

> Phenols are antioxidants found only in plant foods. They have both antioxidant and anti-inflammatory effects on the body.

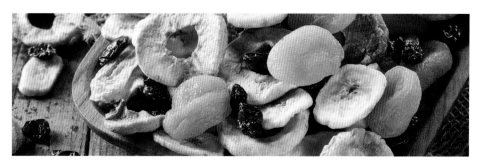

RECOMMENDATIONS:

- Regularly incorporate dried fruits in your diet. Add them to cereals, smoothies, oatmeal, and granola.
- Use dates to sweeten foods like smoothies, oatmeal, granola, muffins, and cakes.
- As much as possible, avoid dried fruits that have added sugar.
- When it comes to raisins, go organic if possible. Traditional grapes, from which raisins are made, are high on the list of pesticide-contaminated produce.[37]

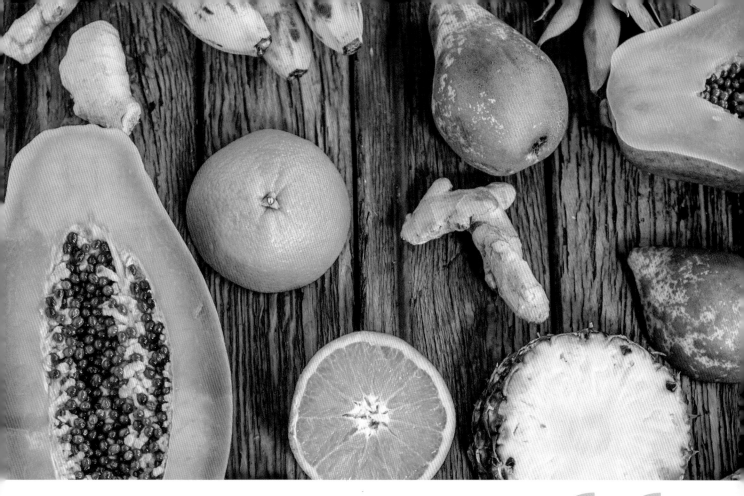

All Fruits

It may seem rather strange to have a section entitled "All Fruits," but it is important to emphasize that *all fruits* provide essential nutrition for the body. Scientific knowledge is often limited by time, money, and manpower. Because of this, research and information is also often limited. Science may say little about the benefits of dragon fruit, guava, and star apple. This, however, may say more about the limits of science than the merits of those fruits.

Because of limited resources, scientists sometimes focus on foods like blueberries, which are well known and more readily available to researchers and consumers in their region. But that does not mean that people in Africa, for example, where blueberries are uncommon, should despair. Fruits, in all their various forms and from all their various regions, offer undeniable benefits in the quest to maintain good health. So whether you are partial to pineapples, sweet on strawberries, or hanker for horned melons, the message is simple. When it comes to fruits, eat them often, eat them raw, and eat as many different varieties as you can.

> When it comes to fruits, eat them often, eat them raw, and eat as many different varieties as you can.

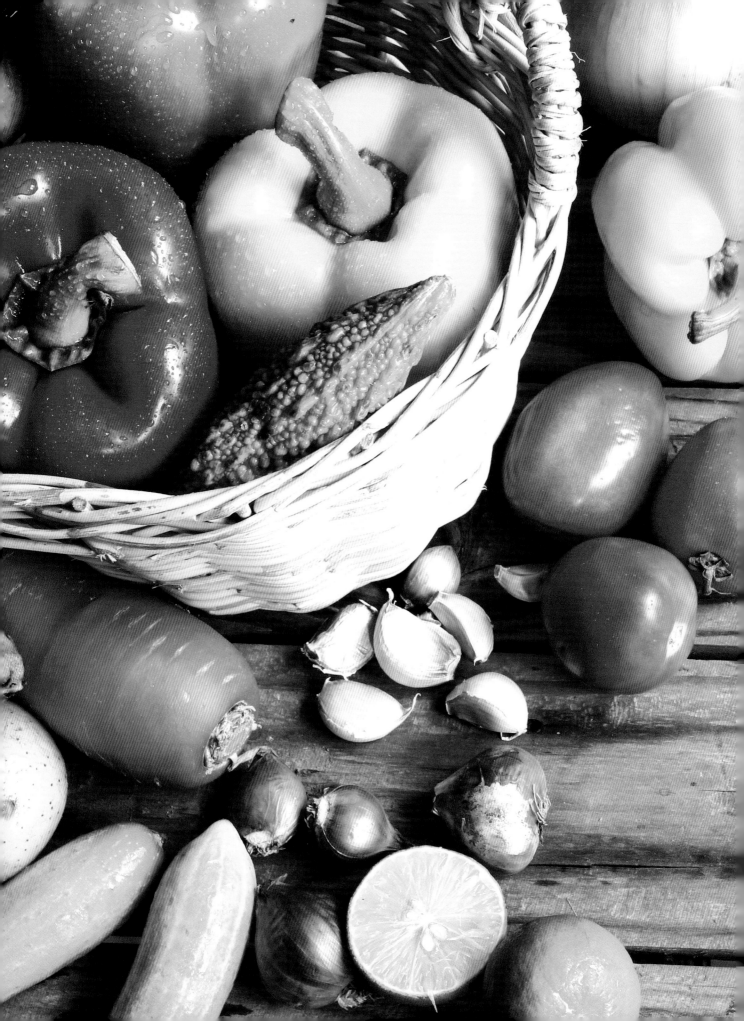

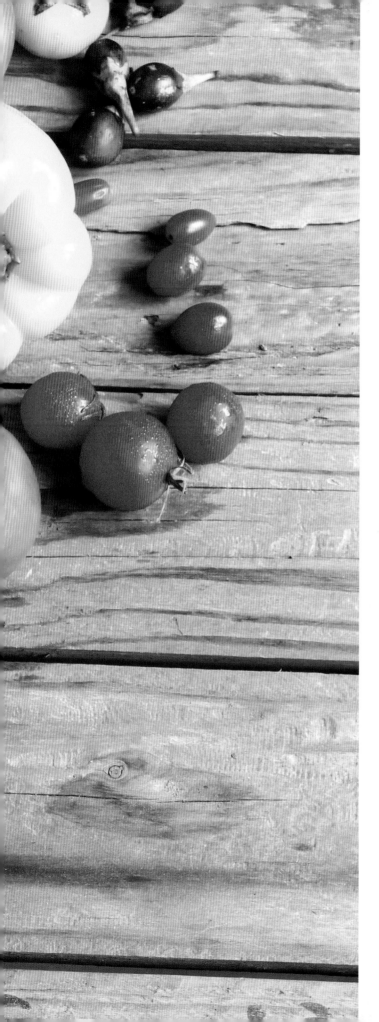

Vegetables

Vegetables are nutritional powerhouses. They are packed with antioxidants like vitamins and minerals. They also contain that all-important plant nutrient, fiber. This is why vegetables play such a significant role in preventing and fighting cancer. One study found that those who eat seven or more servings of fruits and vegetables a day reduce their risk of cancer by 25 percent, and vegetables had the strongest effect.[38] Each daily portion reduced the risk of death by any cause by 16 percent.[39] It is no wonder then that vegetables are such an essential component to good health.

Scientists have studied specific vegetables and vegetable categories to get a better understanding of their health-promoting properties. Still, scientists are far from gaining a full grasp of the varied types and benefits of vegetables. So simply make vegetables from a wide range of categories a regular and abundant addition to your diet.

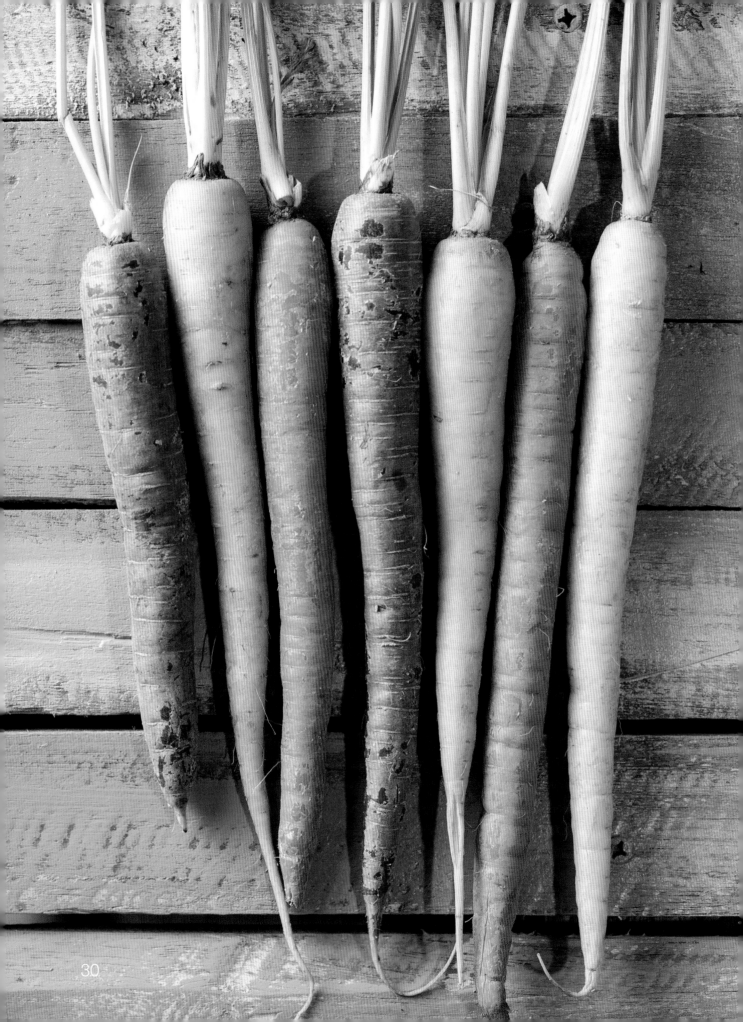

Carrots

From orange to purple to yellow to red and even white, carrots are a richly colored vegetable with benefits that are more than skin-deep. This is because a compelling lineup of antioxidant molecules gives them their beautiful hues. Orange carrots have the ever-popular beta-carotene to thank for their color. Anthocyanins make some carrots purple. Lycopene makes other carrots red. Lutein gives some carrots a pleasant shade of yellow.[40] Carrots also contain fiber, which helps prevent obesity and move waste through the system, capturing and taking carcinogens with it.

Many studies have demonstrated the impact of carrots on cancer prevention and treatment:

- Women who eat raw or cooked carrots as well as spinach (especially raw spinach) have a 44 percent lower risk of developing breast cancer.[41]
- Smokers who do not eat carrots are three times more likely to develop lung cancer than smokers who eat carrots more than once per week.[42]
- Daily consumption of fresh carrot juice protects against the recurrence of breast cancer.[43]
- Women who eat foods containing lutein, alpha-carotene, and beta-carotene are less likely to develop cancer overall.[44]
- Extracts in carrot juice cause leukemia cells to die.[45]
- Consuming beta-carotene may provide some protection against prostate cancer.[46]
- A chemical found in carrots called falcarinol has been found to reduce the risk of cancer development in rats by one-third.[47]

Carrots are a delicious and convenient way to get some of the goodness nature provides. They may be eaten raw or cooked. Indeed, according to one study, properly cooked carrots may supply even more valuable antioxidants than raw ones.[48]

> Women who eat raw or cooked carrots as well as spinach (especially raw spinach) have a 44 percent lower risk of developing breast cancer.

RECOMMENDATIONS:

- Look for ways to incorporate carrots into everyday meals. Put them in sandwiches, blend them in soups, include them in wraps, or eat them all by themselves.
- If cooking carrots, avoid frying and opt instead to steam or boil them whole to maximize their nutritional content.[49]
- Avoid baby carrots. They are simply larger, imperfect carrots that have been shaved down to size to make them more appealing. Like many fruits and vegetables, valuable nutrients are concentrated in carrot skins and the areas immediately beneath, and these are stripped away when processing baby carrots.
- Try carrots of other colors for a little nutrient variety, especially those with a deep purple hue. Purple carrots actually have more than two times the alpha and beta-carotene content of their yellow relatives. They also contain anthocyanins, the same chemicals that give some berries their powerful protective properties.[50]

Beta-Carotene Rich Vegetables

When we think of beta-carotene, we often think of carrots. But carrots are not the only vegetable that contain this important antioxidant. Sweet potatoes and raw spinach contain some of the highest levels of beta-carotene out there. Other excellent sources are pumpkins, squash, broccoli, and green leafy vegetables such as kale, collard greens, lettuce, and mustard greens.

Beta-carotene is important because

- it has antioxidant properties that protect cells from damage. These same properties can also repair damaged cells that might otherwise initiate cancer formation and

- the body converts beta-carotene into vitamin A apart from its well-known benefits in vision and eye health, Vitamin A is essential for a healthy immune system.

Much research has been done on beta-carotene's influence for good health:

- Women who eat more beta-carotene rich foods have a lower incidence of breast cancer.[51]

- Low intake of beta-carotene increases the risk for developing lung cancer.[52]

- Low intake of beta-carotene is associated with increased risk of developing stomach cancer.[53]

- Incidences of tumors in rats fed a carcinogen in cooked meat drop from 58 percent to 32 percent when rats are fed spinach.[54]

It is important to note that beta-carotene is beneficial when we get it through *dietary sources*, not supplements. Beta-carotene supplements do not show a benefit. On the contrary, their use has been linked to increased risk of lung cancer in certain populations.[55]

> Beta-carotene is beneficial when we get it through *dietary sources*, not supplements. . . . On the contrary, [use of supplements] has been linked to increased risk of lung cancer in certain populations.

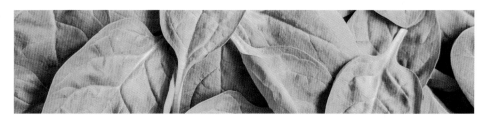

RECOMMENDATIONS:

- Eat two or more servings of beta-carotene rich foods each day. For maximum protection, eat four or more servings. While some of the richest sources are in orange and dark green vegetables, they are also found in fruits such as cantaloupes and apricots.

- Avoid beta-carotene supplements.

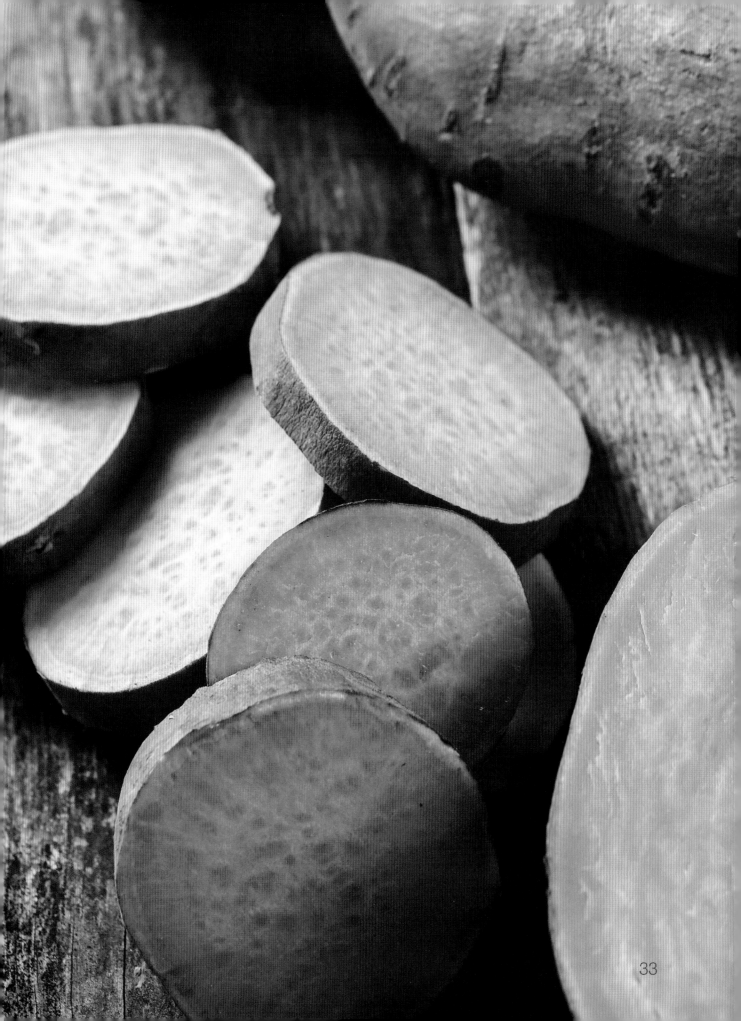

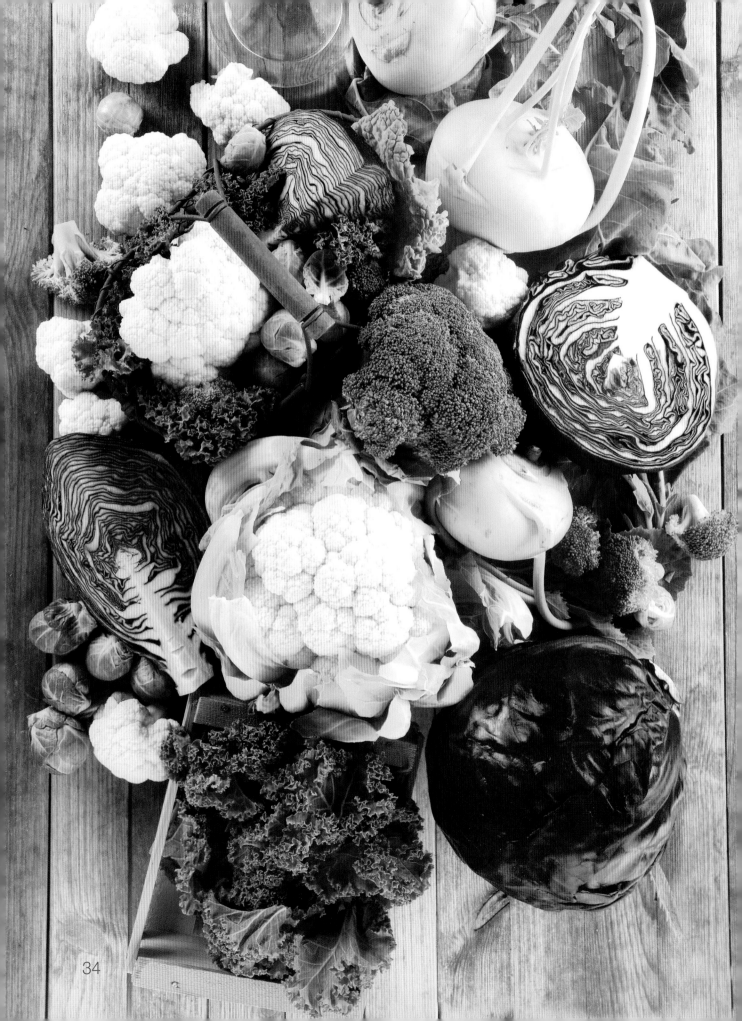

Cruciferous Vegetables

You've probably heard about vegetables like broccoli, cauliflower, cabbage, kale, brussels sprouts, collard greens, and turnips. Maybe you regularly eat some of them. Together, these and other plants form the category of vegetables known as cruciferous vegetables.

Cruciferous vegetables contain substances called glucosinolates, which are converted in the body to other substances like sulforaphane and indoles.[56] What do these do? Here's what the research says:

- Sulforaphane helps quickly clear carcinogens from the body. It triggers the liver to produce enzymes that neutralize substances that cause cancer. It also causes cancer cells to destroy themselves.[57]

- Indole-3-carbinol induces programmed death in various tumors including breast, prostate, leukemia, and colon cancer. It promotes the production of tumor-suppressing proteins and helps regulate estrogen that is implicated in cancers like breast and prostate cancer.[58]

Cruciferous vegetables have a few other things going for them. They are high in:

- **Alpha and beta-carotenes,** which have antioxidant properties that protect and repair cells from damage.

- **Vitamin K,** which reduces inflammation in the body.[59] This is important because inflammation provides an ideal environment for the growth and reproduction of cancer cells. Vitamin K also has antioxidant properties that protect brain cells from oxidative damage.[60]

- **Fiber.** If you eat just 100 calories of cruciferous vegetables, you get 25–40 percent of your daily fiber needs.[61] Fiber helps control weight and moves waste quickly through the body, capturing carcinogens and removing them before they can do damage. Additionally, when fiber is digested by bacteria in the colon, it produces a substance called butyrate. Butyrate inhibits the growth of cancer cells and causes them to die while leaving normal cells unharmed.[62]

This simple group of vegetables provides enormous benefits in cancer prevention and treatment. Studies have found that:

- High intake of cruciferous vegetables significantly reduces the risk of pancreatic cancer.[63]

- High intake of cruciferous vegetables, including broccoli and cauliflower, results in a reduced risk of aggressive prostate cancer.[64]

- Men with prostate cancer who have the highest intake of cruciferous vegetables have a 59 percent reduction in their cancer progression compared with those who eat fewer cruciferous vegetables.[65]

- Intake of cruciferous vegetables among heavy smokers results in a 32–48 percent reduction in the risk of lung cancer. Those who consume more than 4.5 servings of raw cruciferous vegetables each month see their risk drop by 55 percent.[66]

RECOMMENDATIONS:

- Eat vegetables from the cruciferous family five or more times each week to take full advantage of its beneficial properties.
- Try to eat cruciferous vegetables raw. If you need to cook them, minimize cooking time. Cooking reduces some of the mechanisms that convert glucosinolates into cancer-fighting compounds.

The Allium Family

Sometimes referred to as "the stinking rose," garlic is famous for releasing strong and pungent odors when crushed. This is because crushing garlic breaks its cell structures. This sets in motion a process that produces a sulfur compound called allicin.

Garlic belongs to the allium family, a group of vegetables that includes onions, shallots, leeks, chives, and scallions. These vegetables are rich in compounds called allyl sulfur compounds (of which allicin is just one). Allyl sulfur compounds are responsible for the pungent odor distinct to the allium family of vegetables. They have also garnered interest in the scientific community for their anticarcinogenic properties.

Sulfur compounds in the allium family of vegetables have been shown to do the following:

- Prevent cancer cells from multiplying and induce apoptosis (cell death) in cancer cells without affecting normal calls.[67]

- Scavenge radicals and thereby prevent them from damaging cells.[68]

- Increase levels of glutathione, an antioxidant that protects cells from damage.[69]

Additionally, studies show that:

- Women who eat significant quantities of garlic have a 30 percent reduced risk of developing colon cancer.[70]

- Men who eat the highest amounts of vegetables from the allium family significantly reduce their risk of developing prostate cancer compared with those who eat the least.[71]

- Individuals who eat larger amounts of garlic experience a 54 percent lower risk of developing pancreatic cancer.[72]

- Individuals who eat raw garlic at least twice a week reduce their risk of lung cancer by 44 percent. For smokers, their risk is reduced by 30 percent.[73]

- Individuals who eat 20 grams of garlic each day are thirteen times less likely to die from stomach cancer than those who eat less than 1 gram per day.[74]

Certain varieties of onions have greater antioxidant capabilities than others. One study showed that yellow onions had eleven times more flavonoids than white onions, and shallots had six times as much of the antioxidant phenol as sweet (Vidalia) onions. In fact, sweet onions had the lowest phenolic rate.[75]

When it comes to garlic, keep three things in mind to derive maximum benefit:

- Garlic must be crushed in order to produce its sulfur compounds.

- When crushed garlic is allowed to sit for 10–15 minutes, an enzymatic reaction occurs that produces allicin.

- Cooking destroys some of the important sulfur compounds studied for their anticancer benefits. But if crushed garlic is allowed to sit for 10–15 minutes, a greater number of the compounds is retained in the cooking process.

RECOMMENDATIONS:

- Try to eat one clove of garlic every day.
- Crush or grate garlic and allow it to sit for 10–15 minutes before using.
- Keep cooking time to a minimum to retain sulfur compounds.
- Regularly incorporate onions, scallions, and other members of the allium family in your cooking.

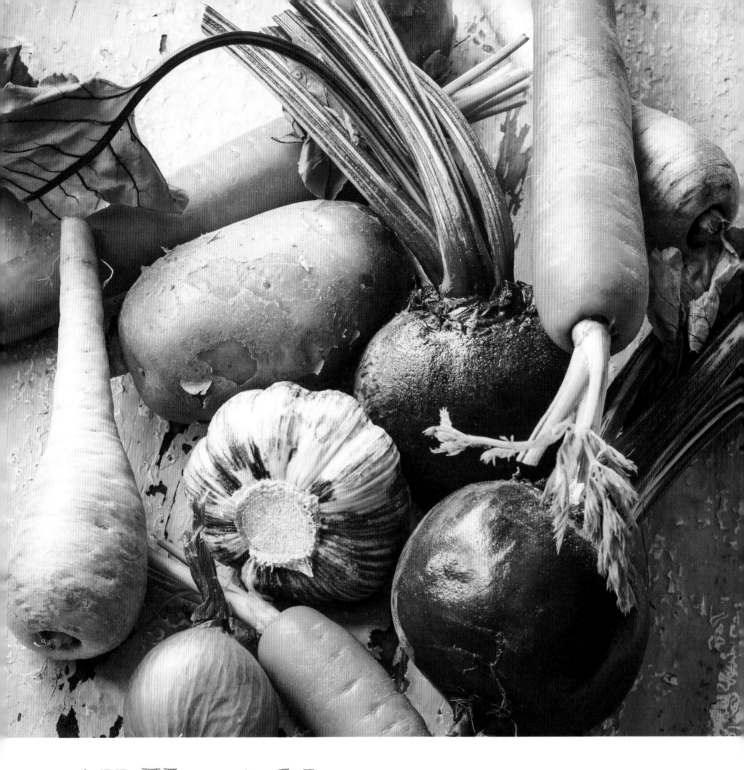

All Vegetables

The world of vegetables is as diverse as the world of fruits. Scientific research is only beginning to scratch the surface in uncovering the nutritional value of the many types of vegetables on our planet. So as with fruits, make it a practice to eat a wide variety of vegetables every day. Your choices do not need to be limited to the vegetables discussed in this book. Feel free to make abundant use of vegetables unique to your culture and climate. Also, unless otherwise mentioned, eat them as close to their natural state as possible—minimally dressed and minimally cooked. If you do, you will reap valuable results.

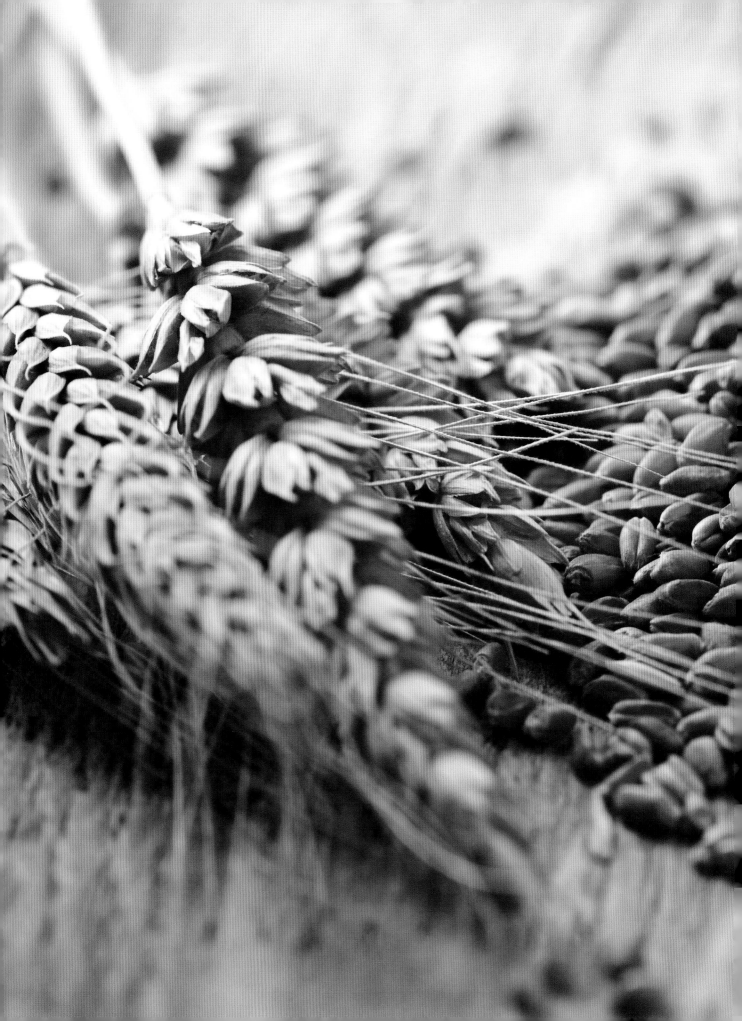

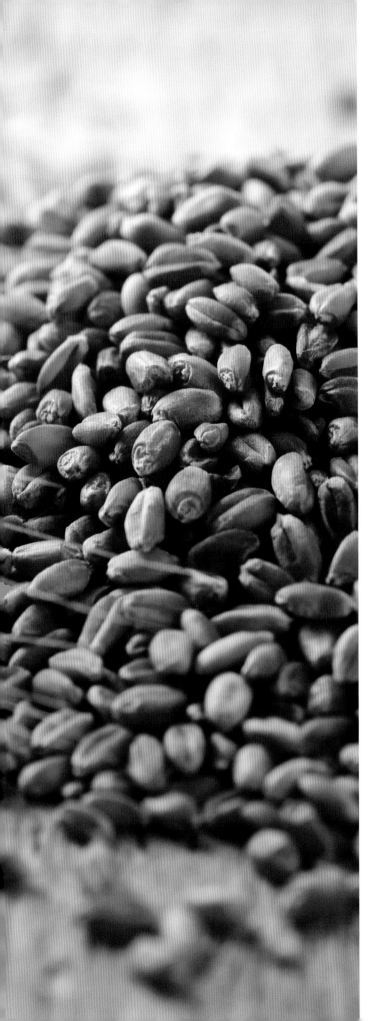

Whole Grains

Naked grains. That's what we get when we buy white rice, white flour, and white pasta. Most people would never think of going outside on a very cold day without proper covering. Doing so can be harmful and dangerous for the body. But when we eat grains that have been stripped of their outer coverings, we do harm to our bodies as well. Why? Because we deny our bodies the dense package of nutrition the whole grain offers.

Whole Grains

Grains like barley, wheat, millet, oats, rice, rye, spelt, and teff are considered whole when they come with *all three of their parts intact*. These parts can be remembered by the acronym **BEG**.

- The **BRAN** is the outer part of the grain that contains most of its dietary fiber. Bran is also rich in antioxidants, including B vitamins and minerals.
- The **ENDOSPERM** is the middle part of the grain and its largest part. It contains carbohydrates, protein, and a few vitamins and minerals.
- The **GERM** is the smallest part of the grain. It has the highest concentration of B vitamins, as well as a few proteins, minerals, and fats.

When grains are refined, the bran and germ are removed, leaving the endosperm. As a result, we lose the fiber, antioxidants, and B vitamins needed to promote health. This is why our bodies *beg* us to eat our grains whole.

So what exactly do whole grains do for the body?

- They provide "concentrated sources of dietary fiber" that improve our gut environment and provide immune protection.[76]
- They are rich in antioxidants that protect against cell damage.[77]
- They contain compounds like *lignans* and *phytoestrogens* that protect against hormone-related diseases like breast cancer and prostate cancer.[78]
- They bind to carcinogens and remove them safely from the body.[79]

Whole grains can bind and remove carcinogens thanks in great part to their fiber content. A number of studies have demonstrated that diets high in fiber also lower cancer risk. They have found the following information:

- Premenopausal women who eat more than 30 grams of fiber a day lower their risk of developing breast cancer by 52 percent compared with those who eat less than 20 grams a day. Fiber from whole grains provides the most protection, a 41 percent reduction, but fiber from fruit is also effective, providing a 29 percent reduction.[80]
- Women who consume the most fiber reduce their chances of getting breast cancer, and every 10-gram increase in daily fiber intake is associated with a 7 percent reduction in risk.[81]
- High intake of dietary fiber, particularly from cereal grains and whole grains, reduces the risk of colorectal cancer.[82]
- Eating whole grains, cereals, and nuts protects against prostate cancer.[83]

RECOMMENDATIONS:

- Eat three servings of whole-grain foods every day.
- Reduce consumption of processed and refined grains such as white rice, white bread, white pasta, and white flour.

> When grains are refined, the bran and germ are removed, leaving the endosperm. As a result, we lose the fiber, antioxidants, and B vitamins needed to promote health. This is why our bodies *beg* us to eat our grains whole.

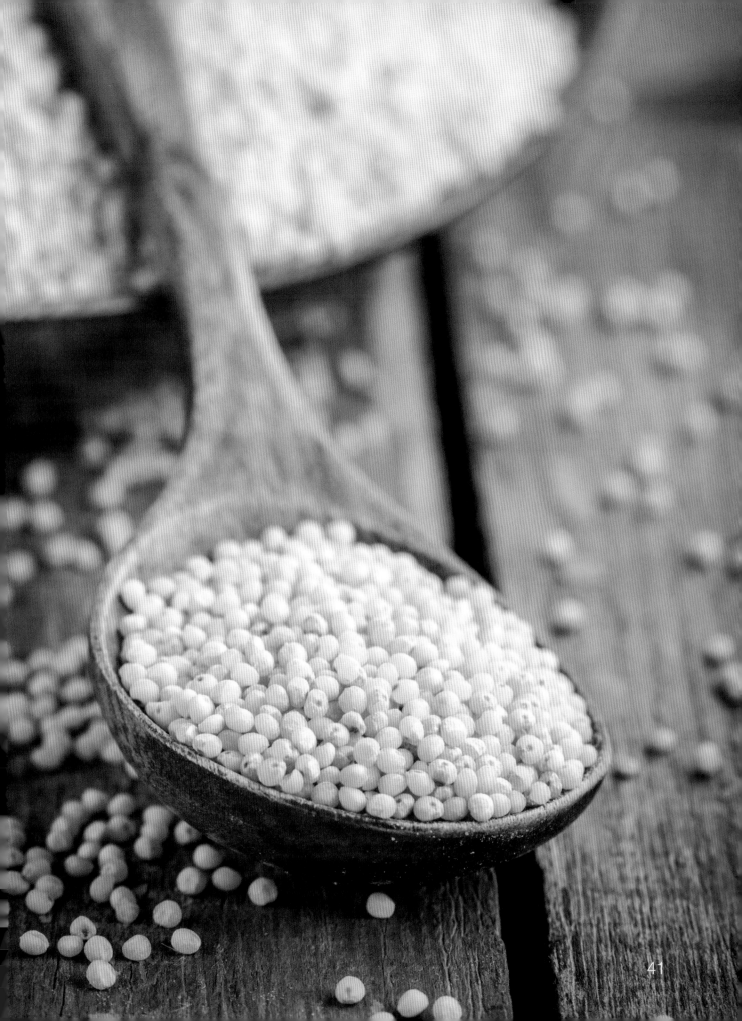

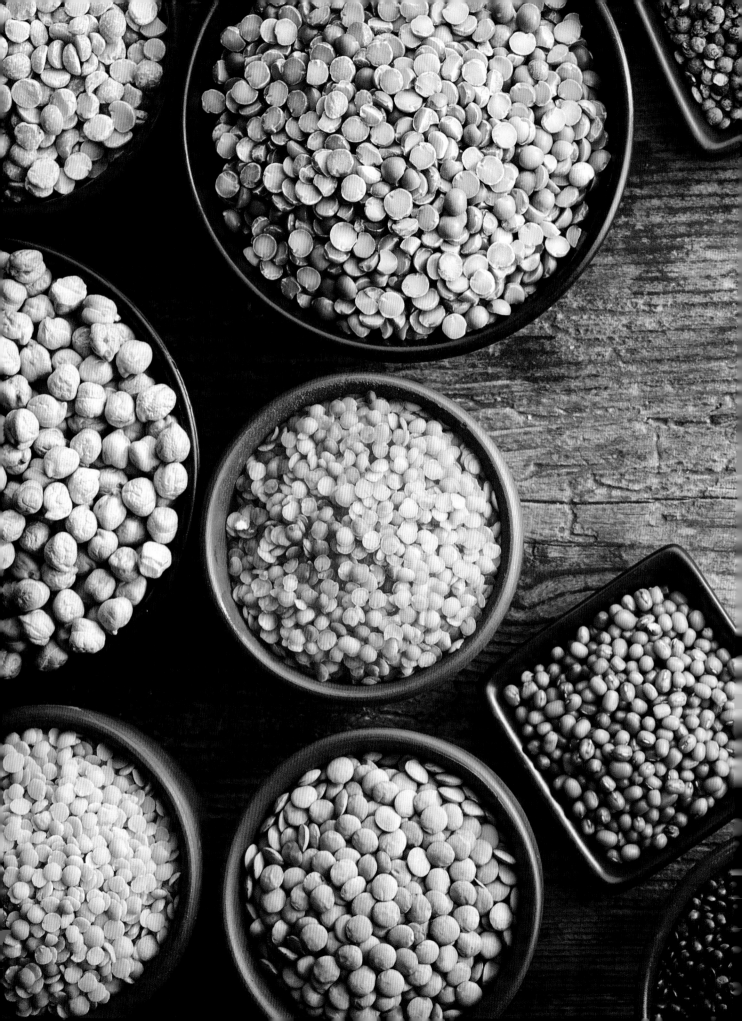

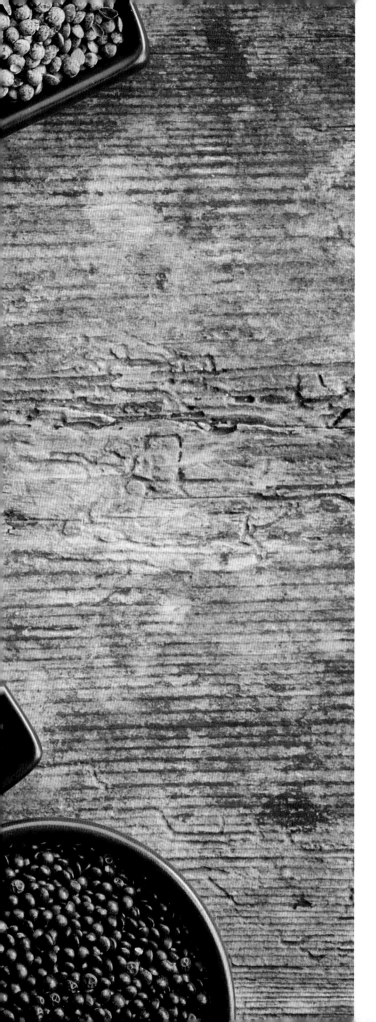

Legumes

They come in different shapes and colors and are a staple of dishes in many countries throughout the world. From Caribbean stewed beans to Cuban black beans to the lentil dishes popular in India, legumes are a versatile, inexpensive, filling, and tasty addition to many diets worldwide. It is wonderful, then, that legumes also have important nutritional components that help protect the body from many diseases, including cancer.

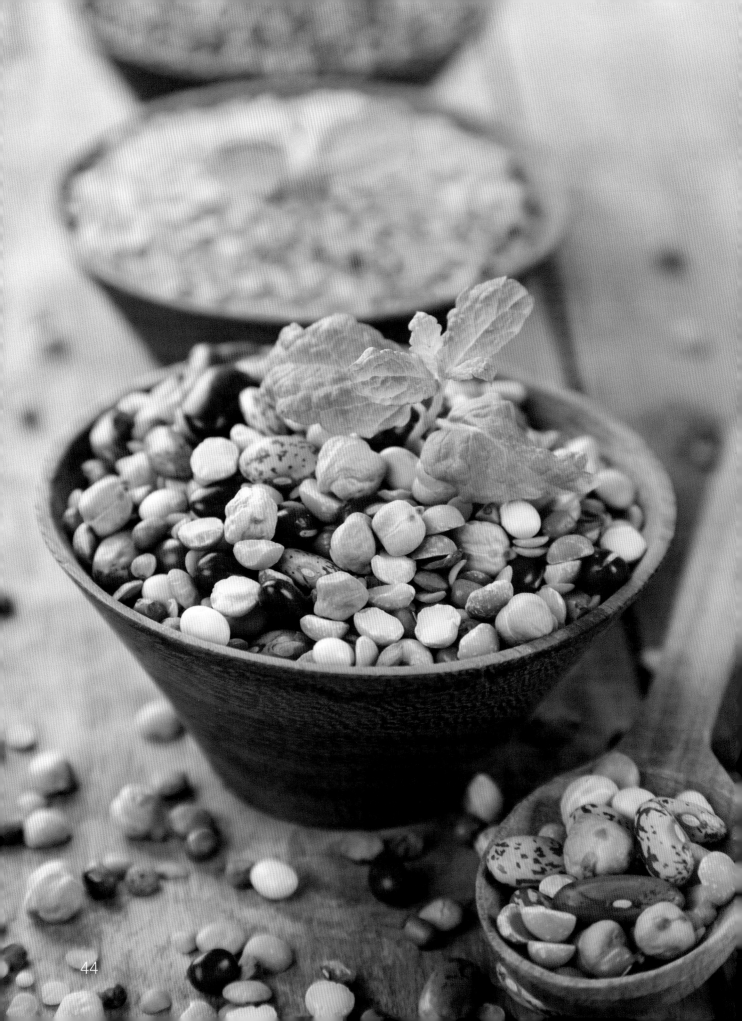

Legumes

You may have heard that beans are good for your heart. The reality is that beans, part of the legume family, are good for much more than that.

Legumes are a category of foods that include *beans* (black beans, soybeans, chickpeas, kidney beans, lima beans), *peanuts*, *peas* (green peas, snow peas, split peas, black-eyed peas), and *lentils*. They are a good source of

- dietary fiber, both soluble and insoluble;
- protein, containing almost as much protein as is found in meat and eggs;
- carbohydrates, an important fuel for our bodies; and
- vitamins, minerals, and other antioxidants.

Legumes play an important role in cancer prevention. Studies have found that the folowing facts:

- Individuals who eat beans more than two times a week have only one-thirtieth the risk of developing pancreatic cancer, compared with those who eat legumes less than once a week.[84]
- People who eat beans at least twice a week reduce their risk of developing colon cancer by 42 percent.[85]
- Women who have the highest intake of allium vegetables and fresh legumes have a 17–26 percent reduction in risk of breast cancer compared with women who have the lowest intake.[86]
- Women who eat beans and lentils at least twice a week reduce their risk of developing breast cancer by 24 percent compared with those who eat them less than once a month.[87]
- Men who have the highest intake of legumes reduce their risk of developing prostate cancer by 38 percent compared with those who have the lowest intake of legumes.[88]

A Word About Soy

Soybeans, part of the legume family, have drawn some controversy in connection with breast cancer research. A couple of studies examining isolated soy components in vitro (in test tubes) and in rat studies seemed to suggest that soy might actually increase the risk of breast cancer. It may be, however, that these studies highlight some of the challenges of scientific research. As Doctor Marji McCullough explains in an article on Cancer.org:

"When concerns about soy are raised, they generally focus on findings from rodent models of cancer which tend to use isolated soy compounds like soy protein isolate or high doses of isoflavones. However, soy is metabolized differently in humans than it is in rats, so findings in rodents may not apply to people . . . until more is known, if you enjoy eating soy foods, the evidence indicates that this is safe, and may be beneficial."[89]

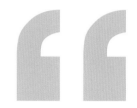

People who eat beans at least twice a week reduce their risk of developing colon cancer by 42 percent.

Soy consumption is linked with lower incidences of hormone-dependent cancers such as breast and prostate cancer because it contains something called phytoestrogen.

In vitro and animal studies are extremely helpful in prompting scientific discovery. However, it is also important to remember that when isolated compounds are removed from their natural context, the outcome may be affected. It is therefore helpful to look beyond studies focused on specific food components and see how foods, in their whole form, influence overall health.

Soy has been consumed in a dietary context for many years and many studies have pointed out clear benefits from its consumption. These studies have found the following:

- Chinese women with higher soy intake have an 18 percent reduced risk of developing breast cancer compared with those that have a lower soy intake.[90]

- North American men who eat at least 1.4 ounces of soy foods a day are 38 percent less likely to have prostate cancer than those who do not.[91]

- Chinese men who consume at least 4 ounces of soy foods daily are half as likely to have prostate cancer as those who consume less than 1 ounce each day.[92]

- Men who drink soy milk more than once daily experience a 70 percent reduction in the risk of prostate cancer compared with those who never drink it.[93]

Soy consumption is linked with lower incidences of hormone-dependent cancers such as breast and prostate cancer because it contains something called phytoestrogen. Excess estrogen in the body unleashes a cascade of events that promote the development of cancer. Phytoestrogens, however, control these activities. They regulate the level of estrogen in the body, protecting against these cancers.

Worldwide, statistics indicate a lower incidence of cancer in general, and breast and prostate cancer in particular, in Asian countries where soy products are regularly and frequently consumed. A 2012 survey of worldwide cancer statistics found that the following:

- In China, a reported 173.97 people out of 100,000 have developed cancer (of any kind). In Canada, the number is 295.72 and in the United States, 317.97.[94]

- Out of 100,000 Chinese, 22.07 are reported to have developed breast cancer. In Canada, it is 79.79 people out of 100,000 and in the United States, 92.93.[95]

- Out of 100,000 Chinese, 5.29 are reported to have developed prostate cancer, compared to 88.9 out of 100,000 in Canada and 98.2 out of 100,000 in the United States.[96]

Food is complicated. A single bean is an intricate mix of chemical substances that interact in ways not readily understood. The body can incorporate the benefits of the bean's intricate interactions when they are eaten whole. When food components are extracted from their natural context, however, unintended consequences may result.

RECOMMENDATIONS:

- Eat at least one serving (1 cup) from the legume family each day.
- Make soy products like soy milk and tofu a regular addition to your diet.
- Eat whole foods and avoid heavily processed foods or food isolates.

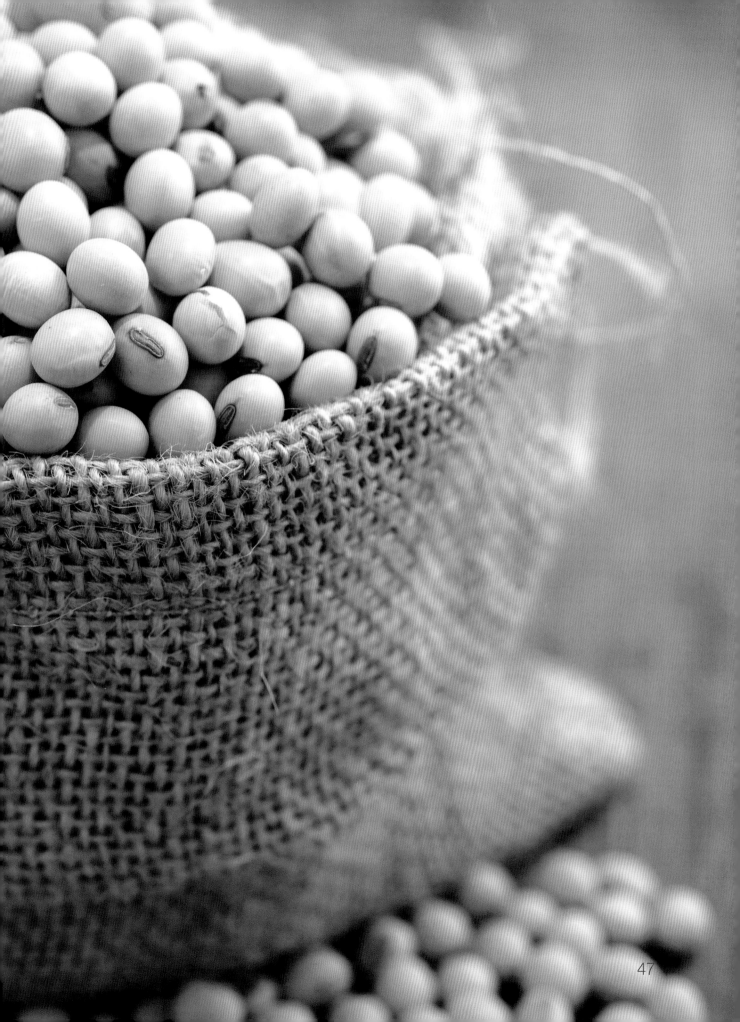

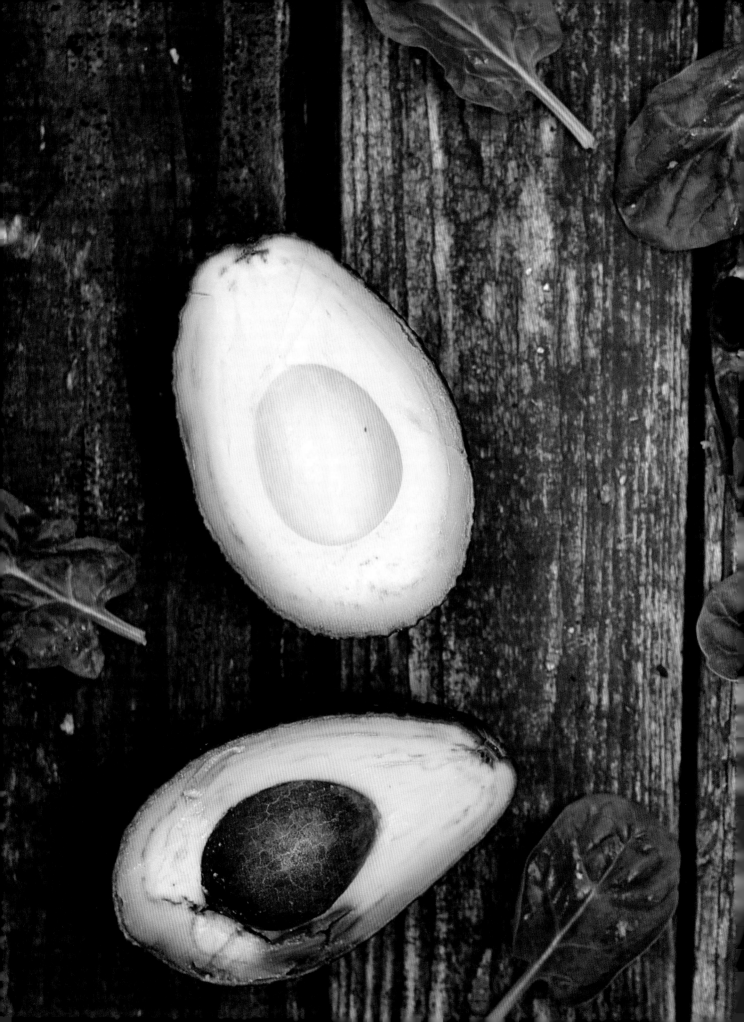

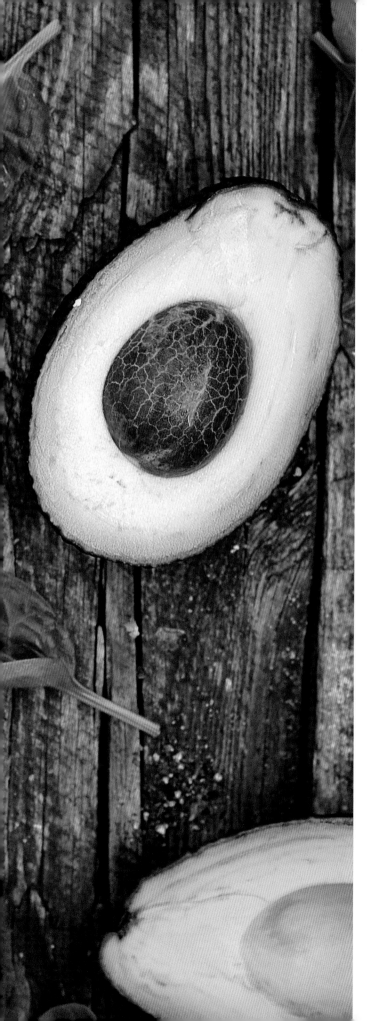

Healthy Fats

Many people hear the word "fat" and want to run to the hills. It's bad for your heart, it's bad for your waist, it's bad for your life—or so many think. But what if I told you that certain types of fat are not only good for you but are essential to healthy living?

Healthy fats, fats derived from plant-based sources, have an important role to play in nutrition. They provide energy, are components of cell walls, help our bodies absorb nutrients, assist in brain and nerve function, and even help lower cholesterol and inflammation. So when it comes to fat, the advice is simple: Don't cut it out. Learn instead to wisely use it.

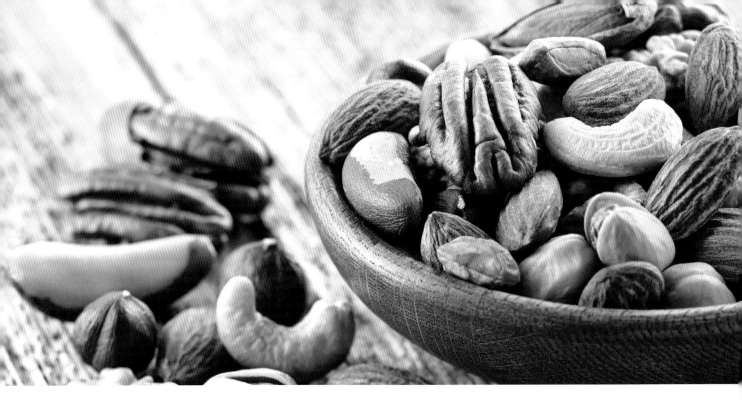

Nuts

Nuts are a rich source of healthy fats, protein, and antioxidants and greatly contribute to overall health. Regular consumption of nuts has been linked to reduced risk of heart disease, type 2 diabetes, and obesity. One large study, following over 115,000 people over a 24–30 year period, found that people who ate a handful of nuts every day were 20 percent less likely to die from any cause.[97]

Nuts may also play a role in cancer prevention:

- Regular nut consumers reduce their risk of dying from cancer by 11 percent.[98]
- Brazil nuts may offer protection against cancer, possibly because of their high selenium content.[99]

Walnuts have received particular attention for their role in cancer prevention and treatment. A review of a number of studies has linked walnut consumption to slowed tumor growth and other protective effects.[100] These have found that:

- Consuming walnuts reduces the risk of developing prostate cancer and causes cancerous cells to grow more slowly.[101]
- Regular walnut consumption can also protect against breast cancer.[102]

> Regular consumption of nuts has been linked to reduced risk of heart disease, type 2 diabetes, and obesity.

RECOMMENDATIONS:

- Finish each meal by eating a small handful of nuts. They will help you feel fuller longer and will provide many nutritional benefits.
- Avoid nuts that have been heavily salted or roasted in oil.

Flaxseeds

Good things come in small packages, and the tiny flaxseed is no exception. Packed with fiber, antioxidants, and omega-3 fatty acids, flaxseeds are also the richest source of an important class of molecules called lignans.

The Phytoestrogen Phenomenon

Lignans are part of the phytoestrogen family. Whole grains, nuts, and soybeans are rich in phytoestrogens, but the lignan content in flaxseeds is off the charts. This is important because phytoestrogens play an important role in cancer prevention.

Estrogen is an important hormone in the body that works, in a way, like a key. Cells in different parts of our bodies contain special "locks" called receptors that are especially made for the estrogen "key." When estrogen fits neatly into these "locks," it opens the door wide to a number of activities that help our bodies function normally. But estrogen can go into overdrive, opening too many doors, causing too much activity, and creating dysfunction that can lead to cancer formation. This dysfunction is at the heart of estrogen-dependent cancers like prostate and breast cancer. But phytoestrogens like lignans can help.

Lignans look like estrogen, act like estrogen, and fit neatly into the locks that are made for estrogen. But they are, in a sense, weaker than estrogen. They open the door to estrogen's activities just a crack, and sometimes, they keep it firmly shut.[103] In this way, they keep estrogenic activities in check and prevent them from getting out of hand. That is why consuming phytoestrogen-rich foods like soy, whole grains, and flaxseeds provides protection against prostate and breast cancer. Here's what the research says about flaxseed in particular:

- Women who eat flaxseed or flax bread experience a significantly reduced risk of breast cancer.[104]
- Postmenopausal women with breast cancer who eat muffins with flaxseed experience increased apoptosis (cell death) of cancer cells.[105]
- Men with prostate cancer who include flaxseed in their diets have significantly lower cancer proliferation rates (the speed at which cancer cells multiply).[106]
- Men who eat a lot of phytoestrogen-rich foods like soy and flaxseed experience a decreased risk of prostate cancer.[107]

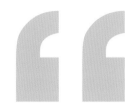

Lignans are part of the phytoestrogen family. Whole grains, nuts, and soybeans are rich in phytoestrogens, but the lignan content in flaxseeds is off the charts.

RECOMMENDATIONS:

- Look for unique ways to daily incorporate ground flaxseeds in your diet. Add them to breads, muffins, waffles, pancakes, granola, cereals, and smoothies.

Olives and Olive Oil

Olives come in a wide range of varieties. There is the yellowish brown Cerignola, the familiar black Mission, the rich green Castelvetrano, and the deep purple Kalamata. The tiny humble fruits of the olive tree are loved worldwide for their unique flavor. They are also prized for their oil. These fruits, part of the much-lauded Mediterranean diet, have also set themselves apart for their significant contributions to health. This is no less so than in the area of cancer.

- Olives and olive oil are rich in antioxidants. Laboratory studies have shown that one of these antioxidants, hydroxytyrosol, keeps human cancer cells from rapidly reproducing and induces apoptosis (cell death).[108]

- Olives and olive oil contain compounds that combat chronic inflammation, a condition that leads to a variety of diseases, including cancer. Oleocanthal, a compound found in olive oil, has anti-inflammatory properties that are similar to ibuprofen, but without its side effects.[109]

Many living in the Mediterranean already enjoy the benefits of a diet rich in plant-based foods, low in animal-based foods, and filled with olives and olive oil. Cancer rates in the Mediterranean are lower than those of the United States, the United Kingdom, and Scandinavian countries.[110] Other studies investigating the relationship between cancer and a diet rich in olives and olive oil have found that:

- Compared to other oils like corn oil, the use of virgin olive oil decreases uncontrolled cell reproduction that causes tumors. It also promotes apoptosis in cancer cells, protects cell DNA, and results in a higher incidence of benign tumors.[111]

- Women who consume higher amounts of olive oil have lower breast cancer risk.[112]

- Women who consume olive oil more than once a day have a significantly lower risk of developing breast cancer, while women who increase margarine consumption significantly increase their risk of breast cancer.[113]

- Consuming olive oil reduces the risk of colon cancer, while consuming meat and fish increases the risk of colon cancer.[114]

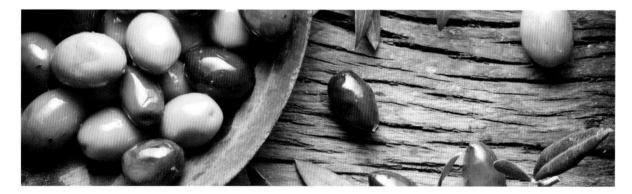

RECOMMENDATIONS:

- Consume olives and olive oil regularly, even daily, to achieve maximum benefit.
- Avoid refined olive oil as its protective nutrients are lost in the refining process.
- Try to incorporate fresh, room-temperature olive oil into your diet. Heat, even at low temperatures, destroys some of olive oil's beneficial compounds. Additionally, cooking olive oil at high temperatures creates harmful substances.

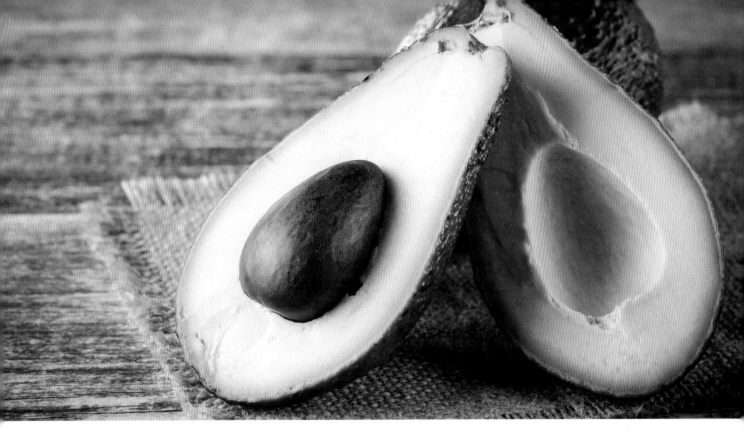

Avocados

Smooth, creamy, with a bright, pleasing color, avocados are a delicious and nutrient-rich food. They have vitamins, minerals, heart-healthy monounsaturated fatty acids, and fiber, and are linked with many cardiovascular benefits. They help reduce total cholesterol and triglycerides and increase levels of healthy HDL cholesterol. But avocados are not just good for your heart. They may also have a role in cancer prevention and treatment. This is because avocados do the following:

- *Have anti-inflammatory properties.* This protects the body from the damage caused by chronic inflammation

- *Contain fiber.* There is about 4.6 grams of fiber in a 2.5 ounce serving (approximately half an average avocado).

- *Contain a number of antioxidants*, including lutein and carotenoids.

- *Increase the absorption of beta-carotene* from tomatoes and carrots by as much as six-fold when eaten with these foods.[115]

- *Contain compounds that inhibit prostate cancer cell growth*[116] and attack acute myeloid leukemia cells, while leaving healthy cells intact.[117]

RECOMMENDATIONS:

- Combine avocados with beta-carotene rich foods like carrots and tomatoes to increase beta-carotene absorption.
- Find unique ways to incorporate avocados weekly in your diet. Include them in salads, use them as a topping for stews, include them in wraps and sandwiches, and incorporate them in desserts such as puddings and homemade ice cream.

Foods That Hurt

Sickness is the vengeance of nature
for the violation of her laws.
—Charles Simmons

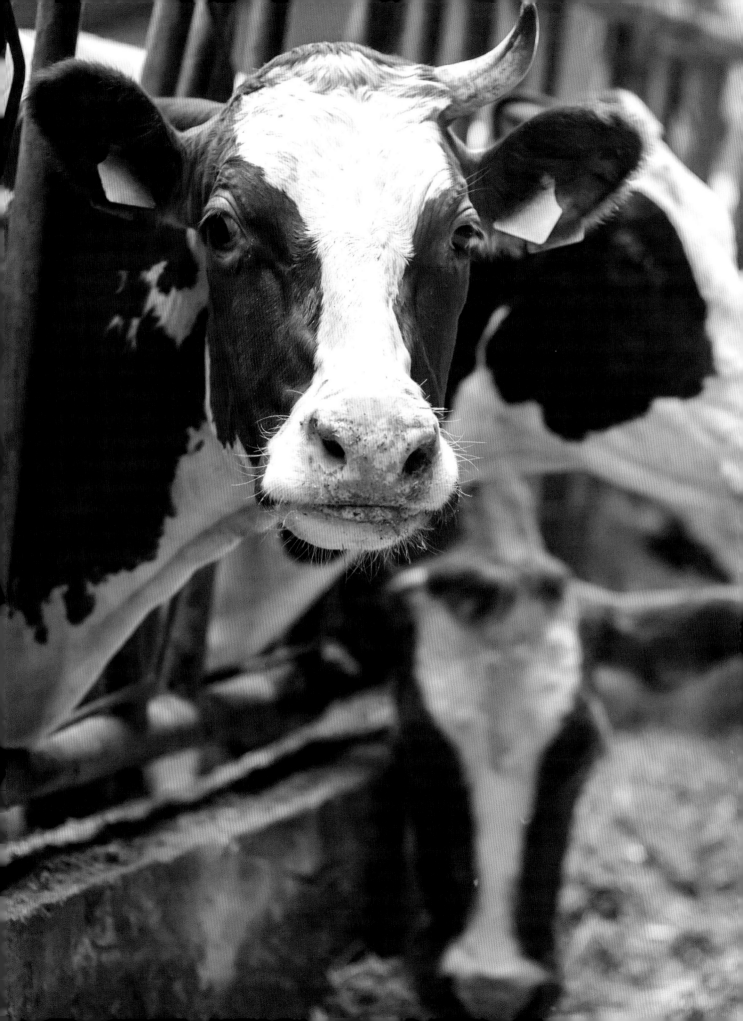

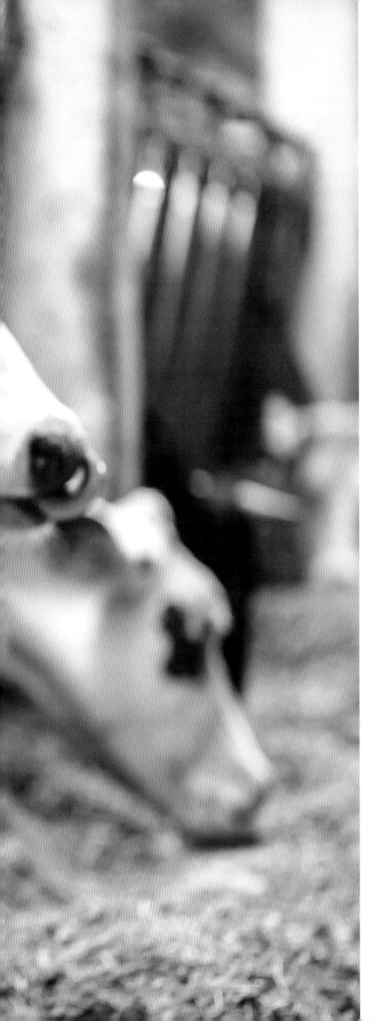

Animal Products

It was 1967, and T. Colin Campbell, a biochemist and professor of nutritional biochemistry at Cornell University, had a problem. At the time, Campbell was in the Philippines working on a project to solve childhood malnutrition. But a troubling issue sidelined his project. Many children in the country were being contaminated by a deadly carcinogen called aflatoxin. The source of the contamination was found in the peanut butter the children often ate. But at this point, the story took a strange turn.

Some of the kids who were affected developed liver cancer even though they were from the "best-fed families" according to Western standards. Indeed, "they consumed more protein than anyone else in the country (high quality animal protein, at that), and yet they were the ones getting liver cancer!"[118]

This puzzling situation caused Professor Campbell to challenge many of the notions he had previously held and strongly advocated in his personal and professional life. Through his research, and that of many others, we better understand how food influences the growth and spread of cancer.

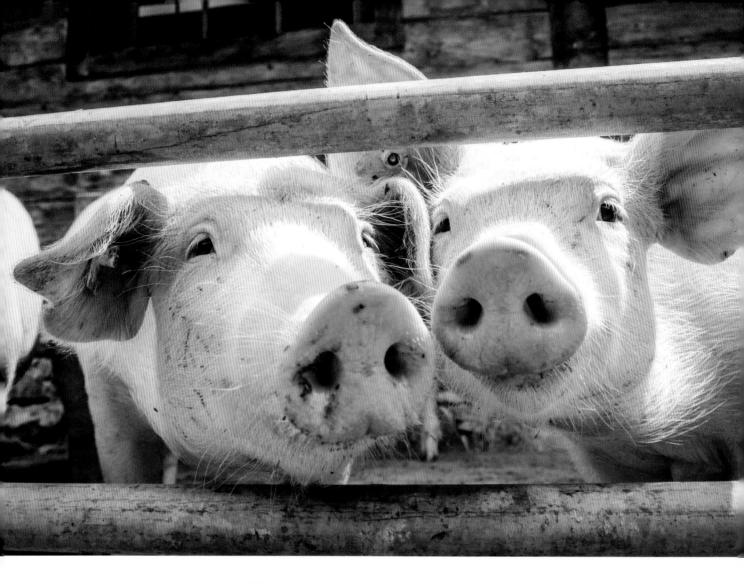

Animal Protein

Sometime after Professor Campbell's experience in the Philippines, he received a grant to study the carcinogen aflatoxin and how it interacts with animal protein. He studied rats infected with aflatoxin and found that

- rats who were given diets containing 20 percent animal protein developed pre-cancer lesions and

- rats who were given just a 5 percent diet of animal protein did not.

Campbell learned that animal protein increases the activity of certain enzymes in cells. These enzymes change the chemical aflatoxin in such a way that it is able to bind to cell DNA and mutate it. Animal protein therefore prompts initiation. It changes a carcinogen in just the right way so that it can bind to cell DNA and cause a dangerous mutation. But plant proteins, even when given at higher doses, do not cause the same cancer-promoting effects as animal proteins.

Animal proteins play another role in carcinogenesis. Insulin-like growth factor (or IGF-1) is a molecule that promotes growth in our bodies and helps us function normally. But diets high in animal protein increase IGF-1 levels,[119] and high IGF-1 levels significantly increase the risk of breast, colon, and prostate cancers.[120] Low-protein diets, however, suppress IGF-1 production.[121]

Meat is defined as the flesh of any animal (including beef, lamb, goat, pork, poultry, and fish). It has been a part of the human diet for many centuries and is prized for its protein content and good taste. But as scientists study the link between diet and disease, a trend emerges. Individuals who frequently eat meat are at a higher risk of developing a number of cancers, including colorectal, breast, stomach, pancreatic, and urinary bladder cancer.[122] On the other hand, those who avoid meat tend to live longer and experience lower incidences of diseases of all kinds, including cancer.[123] This may be because of what meat lacks and what it contains.

Meat lacks many of the beneficial nutrients found in plant-based foods that protect against cancer. It does not contain fiber and is not a good source of vitamins and other antioxidants. It also contains substances that increase cancer risk. Meat contains creatine, a molecule that helps muscles contract. When creatine and the amino acids in meat come in contact with heat, they form a carcinogen called a heterocyclic amine (HCA).[124] When meat is cooked for longer periods of time or at high heat, HCA levels increase.[125]

Meat cooked over an open flame produces another class of molecules called polycyclic aromatic hydrocarbons (PAHs). Certain PAHs are known to be both carcinogenic and mutagenic.[126]

Nitrosamine is another carcinogen that causes tumors to form in the body. It is created when nitrites, which are used to cure meat, react with amino acids in the meat itself.[127] When meat that has been processed in this way is heated, it has a higher capacity to cause genetic mutations.[128]

When it comes to health and cancer risk, animal protein has little going for it and much that can be counted against it:

- Women who eat high amounts of red meat in adolescence or early adulthood have an increased risk of developing breast cancer later in life. A one-serving-a-day increment in red meat is associated with a 22 percent higher risk of premenopausal breast cancer and a 13 percent higher risk of breast cancer overall.[129]

- Women who eat the highest levels of animal protein and fat and the lowest levels of fiber are twice as likely to develop breast cancer as women who eat the lowest levels of animal protein and fat and the highest levels of fiber.[130]

- Men who eat processed meat and red meat cooked at high temperatures have an increased risk of advanced prostate cancer.[131]

- Individuals who consume 5 ounces or more of red meat a day are one-third more likely to develop colon cancer than those who eat less than an ounce a day.[132]

- Individuals who have a high protein intake have a 75 percent increase in overall mortality (death) and a four-fold increase in cancer and diabetes mortality. However, the association between protein and mortality disappears or is reduced if the source of protein is plant-based.[133]

- High consumption of red and processed meats is linked to a substantial increase in cancer in the lower colon and rectum.[134]

- High consumption of red meat increases cancer risk by 28 percent, and processed meat consumption increases risk by 20 percent.[135]

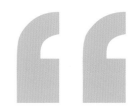

Individuals who frequently eat meat are at higher risk for developing a number of cancers, including colorectal, breast, stomach, pancreatic, and urinary bladder cancer.

Dairy and Animal Fat

Casein, a protein in milk and other dairy products, has been found to promote the development of cell mutations that cause cancer.

Casein, a protein in milk and other dairy products, has been found to promote the development of cell mutations that cause cancer. Returning to Professor Campbell and his research on aflatoxin, the protein he used to test the impact of protein on cancer was casein. So the rats who received a diet with 20 percent animal protein received casein as their protein, and they developed pre-cancer lesions.[136] But Campbell's research is not the only body of evidence to find a connection between dairy and cancer:

- Women diagnosed with early-stage invasive breast cancer who consume high-fat dairy products have a higher risk of dying from breast cancer than those who have little or no high-fat dairy. Women who consume the highest amounts of high-fat dairy have a 49 percent higher chance of dying from breast cancer.[137]

- Men who consume high amounts of dairy products have a 50 percent increased risk of developing prostate cancer.[138]

Dairy may affect cancer risk for a few reasons. First, it contains high levels of estrogen. This is because cow's milk is produced by pregnant cows, and pregnancy is linked to high hormone levels, including estrogen. Estrogen produced by cows does not regulate estrogenic activity like the phytoestrogens found in flaxseeds, whole grains, and legumes like beans and soy. Instead, it promotes estrogenic activity and thereby increases breast cancer risk.[139]

In the case of prostate cancer, dairy may also be risky because of its high calcium content.[140] One study found that high calcium intake, mainly from dairy products, lowers the levels of 1,25-dihydroxyvitamin D3 (more commonly known as vitamin D). This is problematic because 1,25-dihydroxyvitamin D3 is believed to protect against prostate cancer[141] by, for example, inhibiting the rapid growth of cancer cells.[142]

Finally, dairy may influence cancer risk because of its fat content.

- There are significant correlations between dairy and lard fat intake and levels of breast, prostate, rectal, colon, and lung cancer and the saturated fat in these products plays a role in cancer promotion.[143]

- Premenopausal women who eat diets highest in animal fats develop breast cancer at a rate that is one-third higher than women who eat the lowest levels of animal fats.[144]

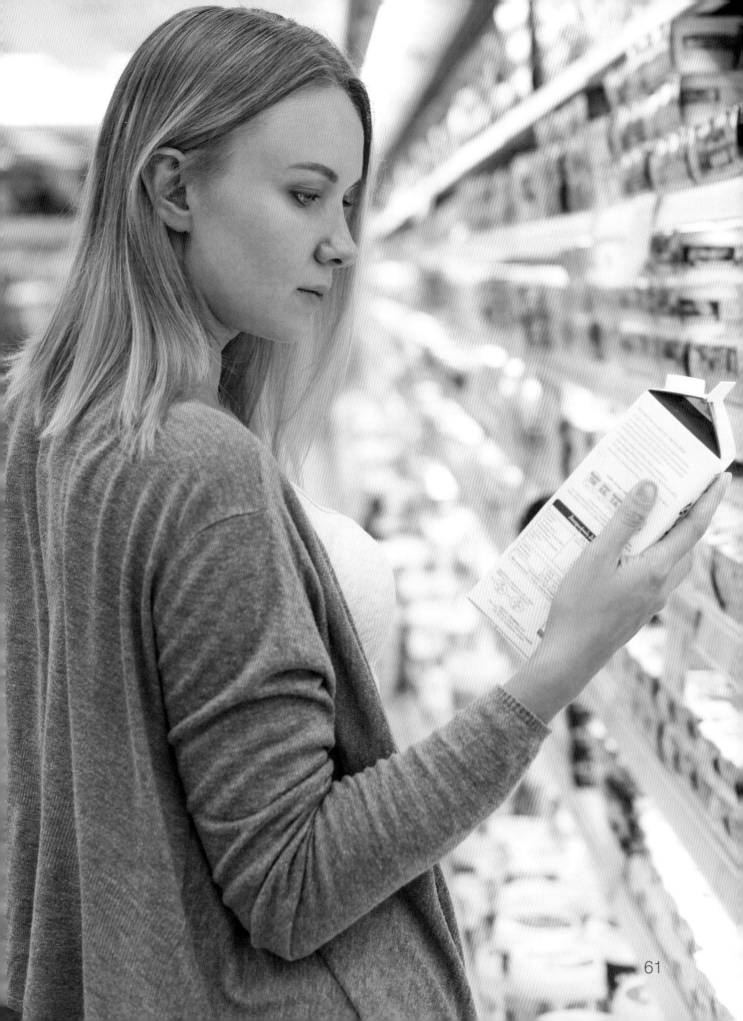

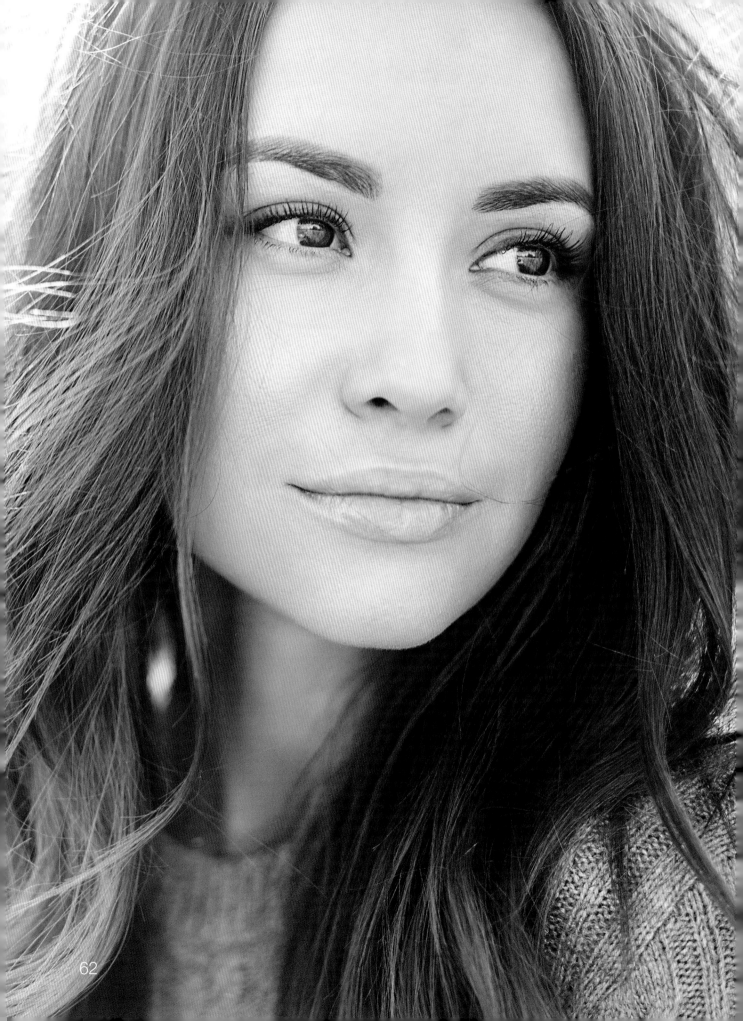

A Reason to Hope

Sometimes scientific research provides reasons for hope, and this is true when it comes to cancer. This is because at various stages of cancer development, changes in diet can result in improvements to health.

One study found that even when our bodies have been exposed to carcinogens, there is a period of delay before tumors begin to develop. During this period, the process of tumor formation "seems to be relatively susceptible to external influences, and it is then that diet appears to exert the greatest effects on tumorigenesis (the formation of tumors)."[145]

But even after tumors have formed, there is still hope. In Professor Campbell's research on aflatoxin, some of the rats who were given the 20 percent animal protein diet and developed liver cancer tumors had their diets switched to a low-protein (5 percent) diet halfway through the experiment. These rats then experienced 35–40 percent less tumor growth than those who were maintained on the high-protein diet.[146]

At any stage of the game, whether the thought of cancer is far from your mind or whether you are in the middle of treatment for the disease, changing the way you eat may prove helpful in the fight for health and life.

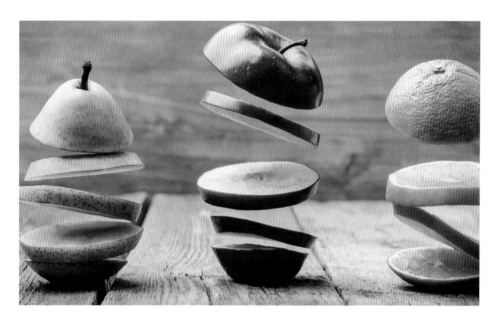

> At any stage of the game, whether the thought of cancer is far from your mind or whether you are in the middle of treatment for the disease, changing the way you eat may prove helpful in the fight for health and life.

RECOMMENDATIONS:

- Reduce or, ideally, eliminate animal proteins from the diet.
- If meats are used, do not cook them at high temperatures or over an open flame.
- Reduce or, ideally, eliminate dairy from the diet, particularly high-fat dairy products.
- Eliminate animal fat from the diet.

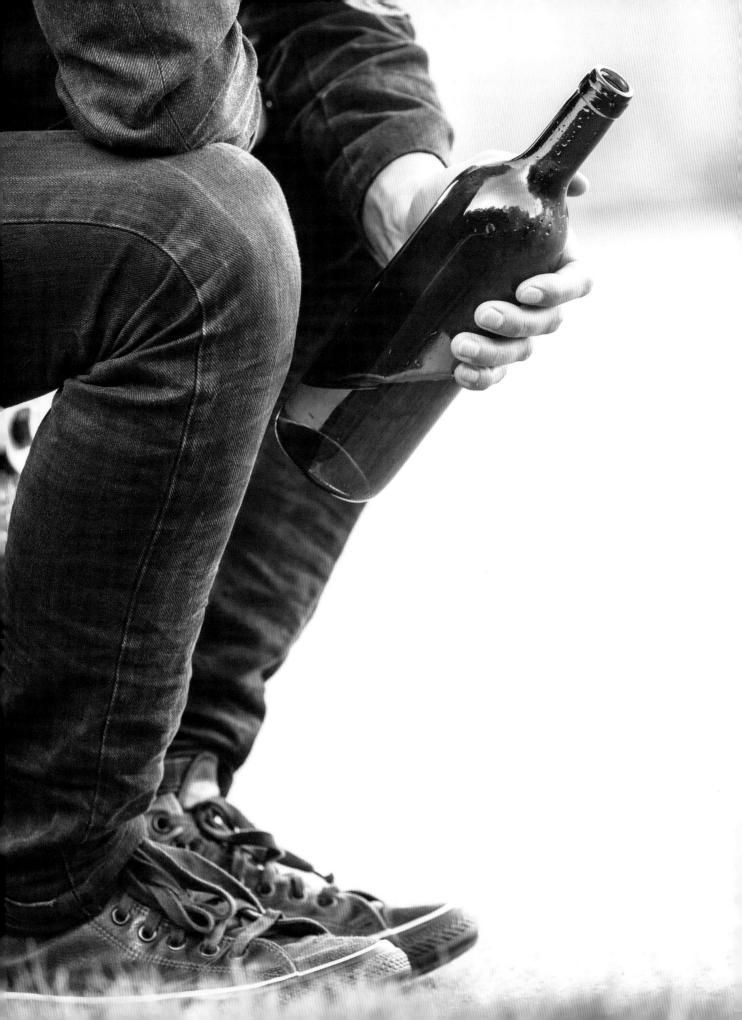

Alcohol

Alcohol use has a long and storied history in human society. It is associated with tradition, ritual, celebration, and the warmth of social gatherings. But ever since humans first learned to ferment and distill, they have discovered that alcohol has a dark side. It is often behind some of the most hateful and violent crimes of our society. Its use negatively affects the well-being of children and adults alike. Whole communities have been devastated by it. What's more, research is discovering that its use, even in moderation, wreaks havoc on our health.

According to the latest statistics, 89.7 percent of Canadians have used alcohol at least once in their lifetimes, and 78 percent have used it in the last year.[147] In the United States, 86.8 percent of adults eighteen or older have had a drink in their lifetimes and 70.7 percent have had a drink in the last year.[148] Alcohol is, without question, a popular beverage not only in North America, but worldwide. But the use of alcohol comes at a cost.

The World Health Organization's 2014 Global Status Report on Alcohol and Health found that alcohol consumption affects cancer development worldwide. Thirty percent of worldwide cases of oral cavity and pharynx cancer, 22 percent of esophageal cancer, 12 percent of liver cancer, 10 percent of colorectal cancer, 8 percent of breast cancer, and 4 percent of pancreatic cancer were attributed to alcohol consumption.[149] So why does alcohol increase cancer risk?

- Alcohol generates free radicals and a molecule called acetaldehyde (AA). Free radicals cause damage to cells, and AA is a carcinogen that binds to DNA and causes mutations.[150]
- Alcohol destroys folate,[151] which plays a significant role in cancer prevention. For example, folate helps produce molecules that repair DNA.[152]
- Alcohol increases the levels of estradiol,[153] an estrogen molecule. High levels of estradiol have been linked to breast cancer risk.[154]

Some advocate light drinking as safe and even potentially beneficial. When it comes to cancer, however, studies show that even light drinking is risky. One study found that light drinking increased the risk of oropharyngeal cancer, esophageal squamous cell carcinoma, and female breast cancer. Five thousand deaths from oropharyngeal cancer, twenty-four thousand from esophageal squamous cell carcinoma, and five thousand deaths from breast cancer were all estimated to be attributed to light drinking.[155]

A Word About Wine

Several studies that examine the benefits of wine on cardiovascular and overall health point to its high phenol content, particularly the antioxidant resveratrol. The trouble is that wine comes with benefits that can be found elsewhere but with risks that are all its own. The resveratrol and other antioxidants found in wine are found in fresh grapes and pure grape juice. These foods do not contain the cancer risks that come with consuming alcohol. Indeed, according to the American Institute for Cancer Research, "[Because of] convincing evidence that alcohol is associated with increased risk for cancers of the mouth, pharynx and larynx, esophagus, breast (pre- and postmenopausal) and colon and rectum (in men), wine is not a recommended source of resveratrol."[156]

> Some advocate light drinking as safe and even potentially beneficial. When it comes to cancer, however, studies show that even light drinking is risky.

RECOMMENDATIONS:

- Avoid the use of alcohol.

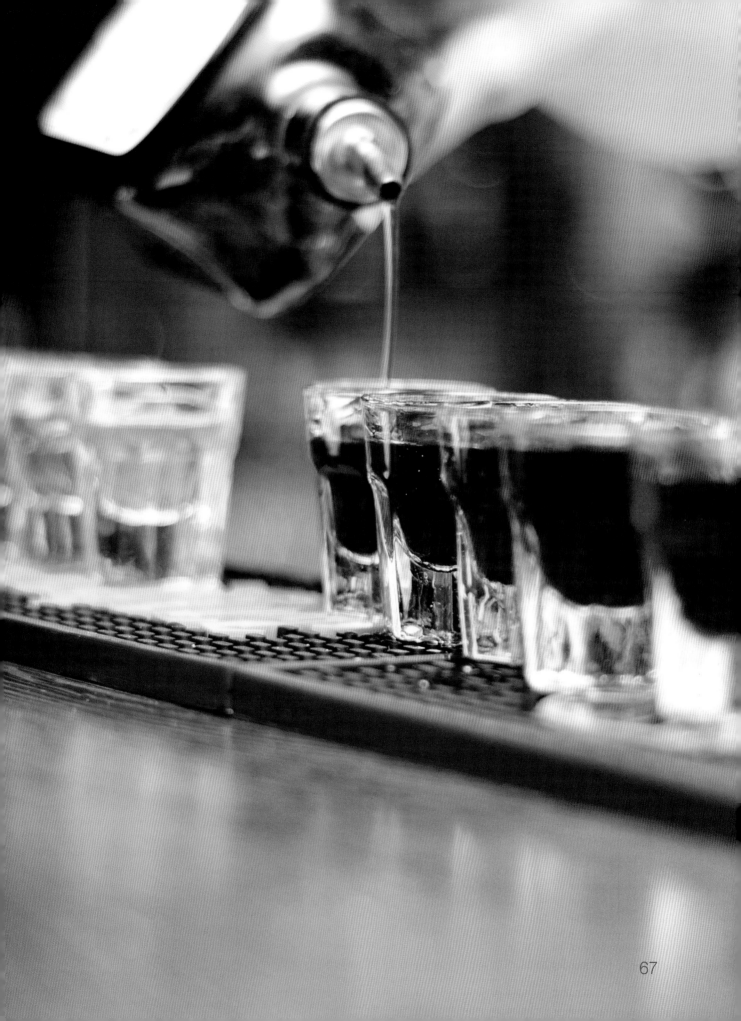

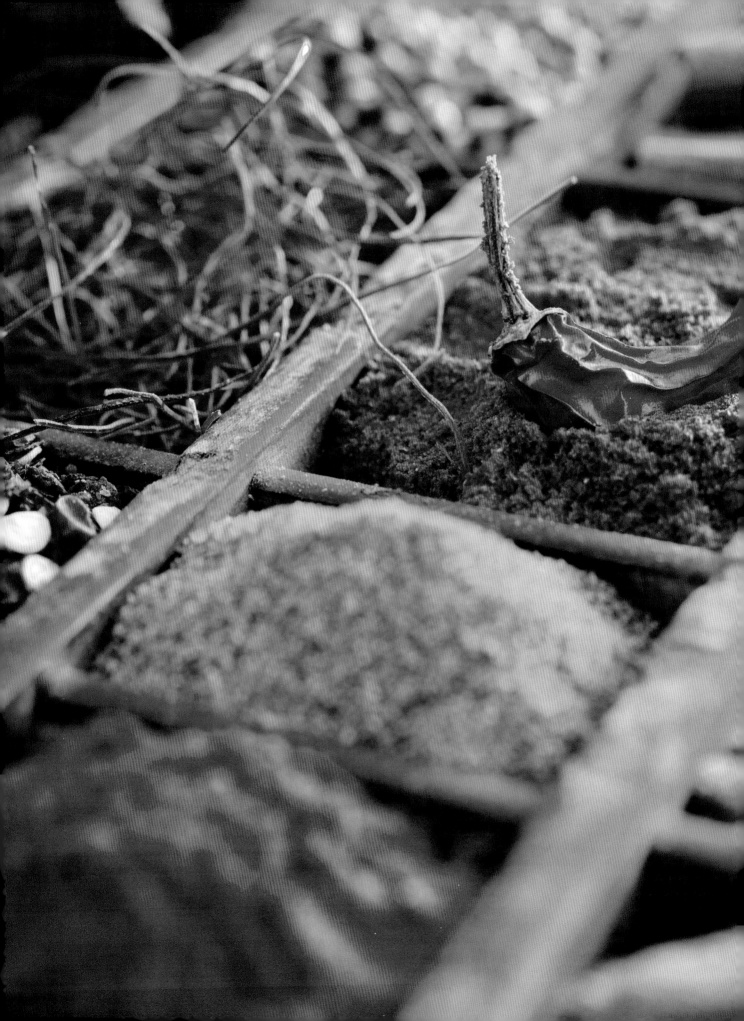

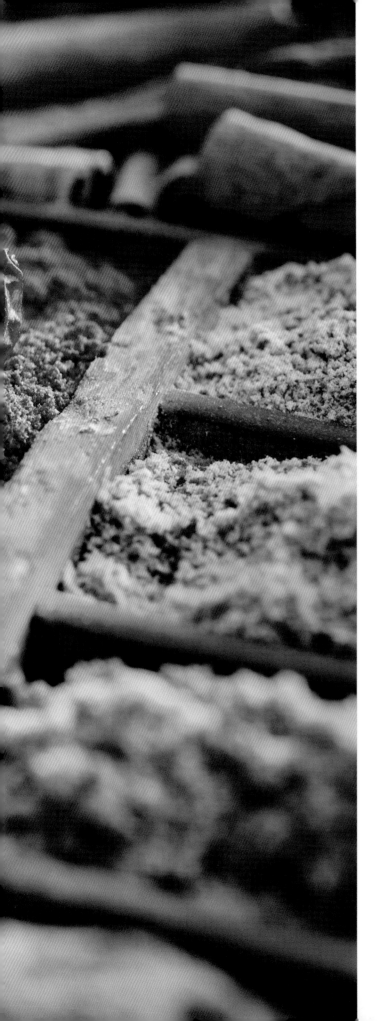

Sugar, Salt, and Spices

Sugar and spice and everything nice—or so the saying goes. And indeed flavor, whether the sweetness of sugar, the savoriness of salt, or the interest of herbs and other seasonings, lend food flavor that many value.

When it comes to health, flavor is important. Healthy food ought to taste good. Still, flavor should never come at the expense of health. When it comes to sugar, salt, and spice, wisdom and moderation in their use will help ensure that food not only tastes good but is good for us too.

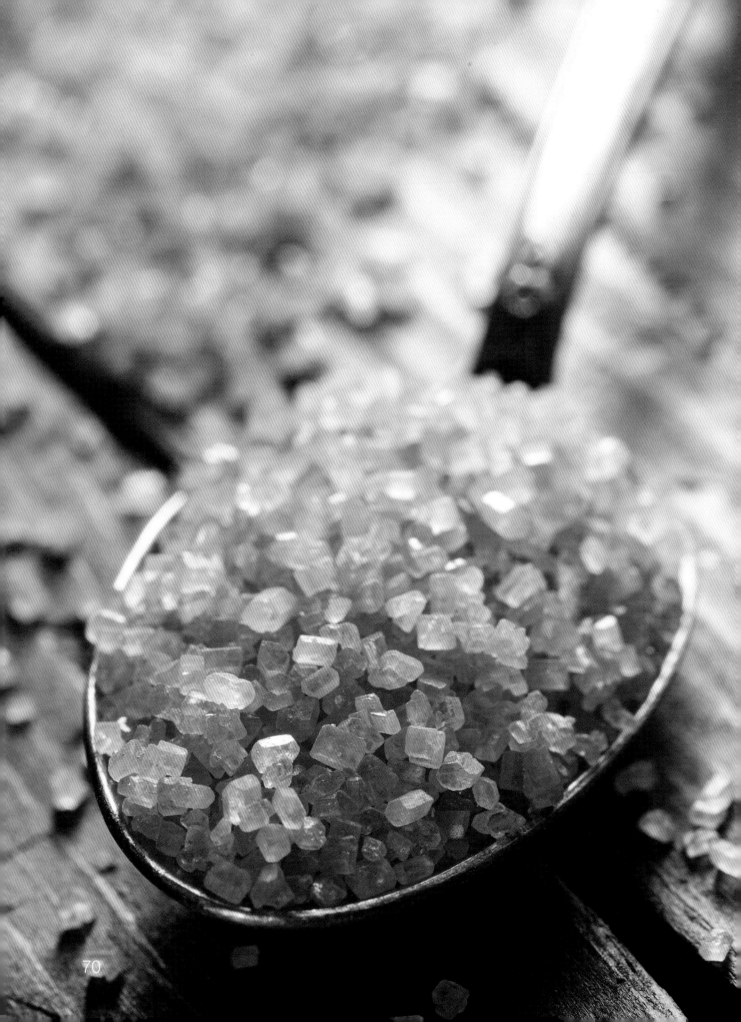

Sugar

Stroll through the grocery aisles to read a few food labels, and you will see that sugar is a popular addition to many foods, from stews to sauces to canned vegetables. The trouble is that the sugar content quickly adds up when sugary foods like sodas, cookies, and cakes are added to the mix.

Consuming excess added sugars is linked to a number of health complications, from diabetes to obesity to dementia to cancer.

- Individuals who consume high amounts of added sugars have increased risk of developing pancreatic cancer.[157]
- Diets high in simple sugars increase the risk of colon cancer.[158]
- There is a high correlation between breast cancer mortality and sugar consumption among older women.[159]

The pancreas produces the insulin that transports sugar into our cells. When we consume excess sugar, we put additional strain on our pancreas. The more sugar we eat, the greater the demand for insulin and the greater the risk of decreasing sensitivity to insulin.[160] This cycle increases the risk of both pancreatic[161] and breast cancer.[162] Excess sugar may also play a role in increased cancer risk because consuming excess sugar often leads to obesity, and obesity is a high risk factor in cancer development.

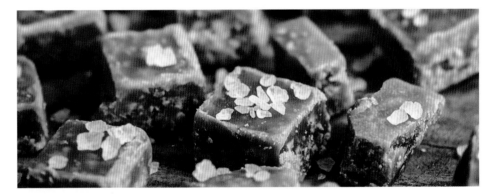

> Consuming excess added sugars is linked to a number of health complications, from diabetes to obesity to dementia to cancer.

RECOMMENDATIONS:

- Limit your intake of added sugars to 6 teaspoons a day for women and 9 teaspoons a day for men. Added sugars include white sugar, honey, maple syrup, brown sugar, and agave syrup.
- Enjoy foods such as fruits and certain vegetables that are a natural source of sweetness.
- Incorporate natural, whole-fruit sweeteners such as dates and raisins into oatmeal, smoothies, and other foods, and use them to replace some of the sugar in recipes for items, such as cakes and muffins.
- Read food labels and monitor the amount of added sugars you consume in the foods you buy.
- Cook your own food so you can control the amount of sugar you put into it.

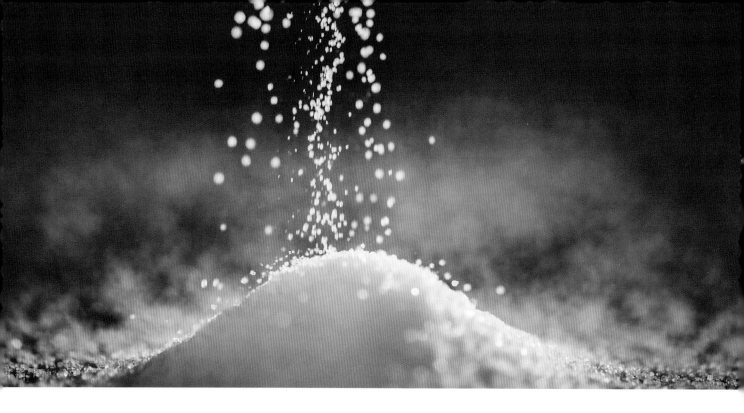

Salt

Many know that consuming excess salt promotes cardiovascular diseases such as high blood pressure and stroke. But the habit of eating too much salt causes problems that go way beyond the heart. It has been linked with obesity, osteoporosis, asthma, kidney disease, fluid retention, and cancer.[163]

Stomach cancer is the cancer most associated with the consumption of excess salt. Salt plays a role in the development of this particular cancer for a number of reasons:

- It causes gastritis, which is the inflammation of the stomach linings.

- It increases damage done by stomach carcinogens.

- It destroys the mucous barrier. This causes inflammation, damage, and degeneration and also makes the stomach more susceptible to carcinogens in food.[164]

Excess salt intake has real-life impact on the prevalence of cancer:

- Individuals with high salt intake have a significant risk of developing gastric cancer.[165]

- Individuals with the highest levels of salt intake experience higher incidences of gastric cancer than those with the lowest levels of salt intake.[166]

RECOMMENDATIONS:

- Limit consumption of sodium to no more than 1,000–1,500mg per day. That's more or less equivalent to ½ teaspoon of regular table salt each day.
- Read food labels to monitor how much sodium is in the food you buy.
- Avoid processed and prepared foods and high-salt foods like chips, pretzels, and fries.
- Cook your own food when possible so you can control the amount of salt you put in it.
- Salt your food at the end of cooking. This often leads to the use of less salt to achieve good flavor.

Spicy Foods

From soups to stews to casseroles, you will be hard-pressed to find a savory recipe that does not include black pepper and other spices. Hot sauce, chili peppers, and curry blends are common and popular go-to methods of adding interest and kick to foods. These days, it seems a taste for heat is all the rage and for some individuals, the spicier the better.

Unfortunately, a tendency to reach for spices has been linked to an increased risk of developing certain cancers. Studies have found that:

- Those who consume very spicy foods and have diets high in chili have a greater risk of developing esophageal cancer.[167]

- Individuals who consume spicy foods and high amounts of chili are at greater risk of developing stomach cancer.[168]

- Individuals who have a preference for spicy foods have a nearly two-fold increase in risk of laryngeal cancer.[169]

- Esophageal cancer is more frequent in Indian populations in several parts of the world, and "the indiscrete use of spices" may explain why risk of developing esophageal cancer is significantly higher in these populations.[170]

Chili peppers contain a compound called capsaicin. This compound has received specific attention in scientific research and is the subject of some controversy. Some studies identify capsaicin as a carcinogen. In one laboratory study, for example, topical application of capsaicin produced skin cancer.[171] In another study, rats were given capsaicin over the course of their lifetimes and as a result, 22 percent of the females and 14 percent of the males developed tumors.[172] On the other hand, some laboratory studies have found that human cancer cells treated with capsaicin experienced apoptosis (cell death).[173]

Because of conflicting laboratory studies, the jury is out about whether capsaicin helps or hurts. But human studies demonstrate a correlation between the consumption of spicy foods, such as chili peppers, and an increased risk of developing various cancers. Perhaps like red wine, the potential risks of consuming spicy foods outweigh the potential benefits of spice compounds like capsaicin. This is especially true since some of the beneficial compounds in spices can be found in other, safer foods.

> Human studies demonstrate a correlation between the consumption of spicy foods, such as chili peppers, and an increased risk of developing various cancers.

RECOMMENDATIONS:

- Limit or completely avoid the use of hot spices in cooking.
- Use ingredients like onions and garlic and herbs to season food and enhance flavor.

Recipes

Eat food. Not too much. Mostly plants.
—Michael Pollan

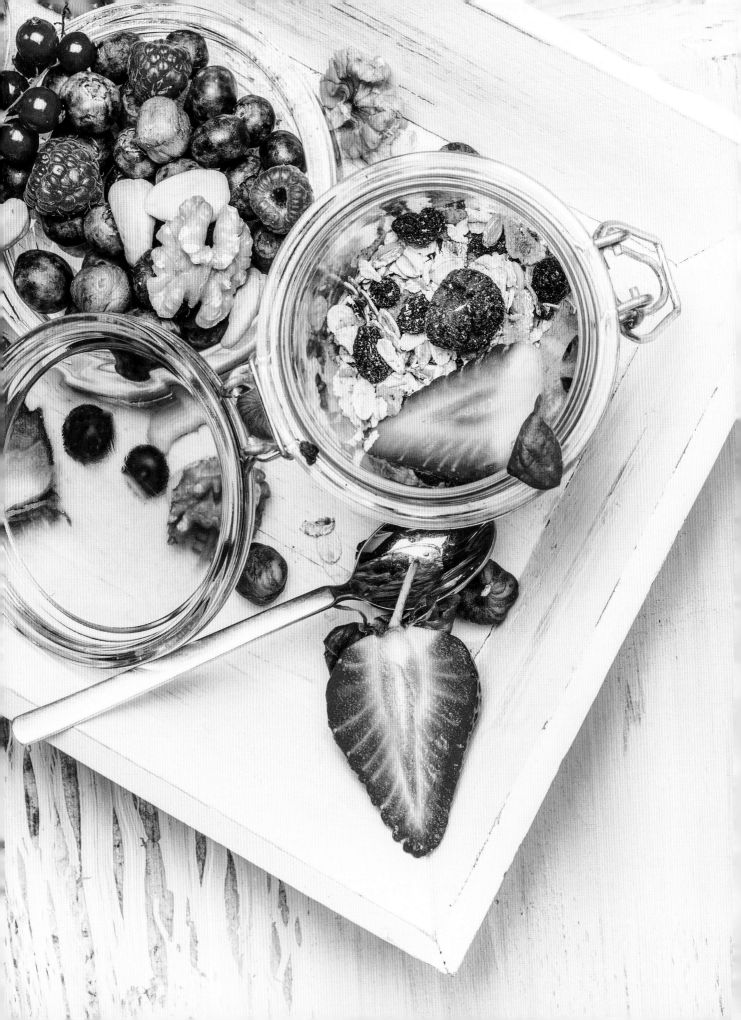

Breakfast

Pumpkin French Toast

Steel-Cut Oats

Berry Waffles

Granola

Nut Milk

Multigrain Flax Bread

Very Berry Smoothie

Tofu Veggie Scramble

BREAKFAST

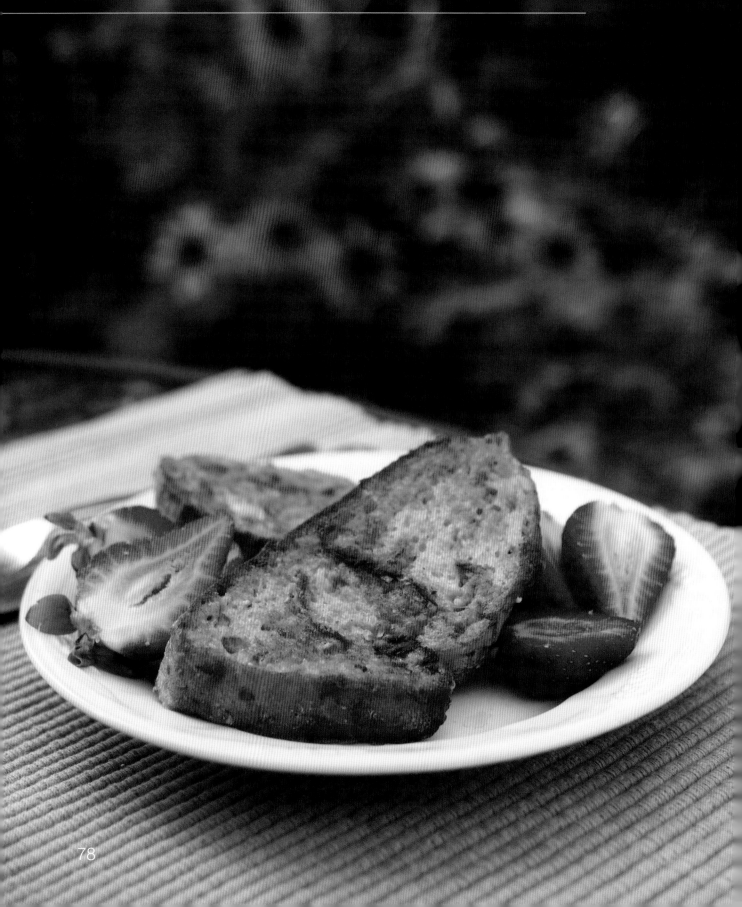

Pumpkin French Toast

INGREDIENTS

- ½ cup pumpkin puree
- 1 cup unsweetened soy milk
- 2 teaspoons maple syrup
- 1 teaspoon vanilla extract
- 8 slices whole-grain bread (preferably a bit stale)

INSTRUCTIONS

1. In a shallow bowl, whisk together pumpkin puree, soy milk, maple syrup, and vanilla. Dunk both sides of bread into mixture.

2. In a lightly sprayed nonstick skillet, cook each side of the bread for 3 to 5 minutes on medium heat, or until each side is golden brown. Makes 4 servings.

SERVING SIZE	TOTAL FAT	CHOLESTEROL	TOTAL CARBS	SUGARS
153 g (2 slices)	2.6 g	0 mg	29.0 g	6.7 g
CALORIES	**SATURATED FAT**	**SODIUM**	**DIETARY FIBER**	**PROTEIN**
180	0.6 g	277 mg	4.8 g	9.2 g

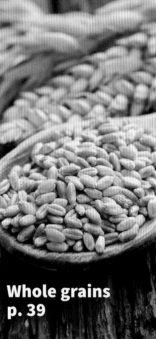

Whole grains p. 39

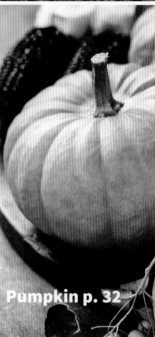

Pumpkin p. 32

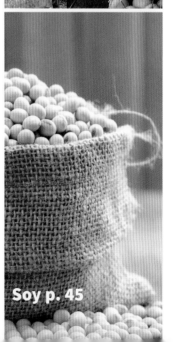

Soy p. 45

Cancer-Fighting Ingredients

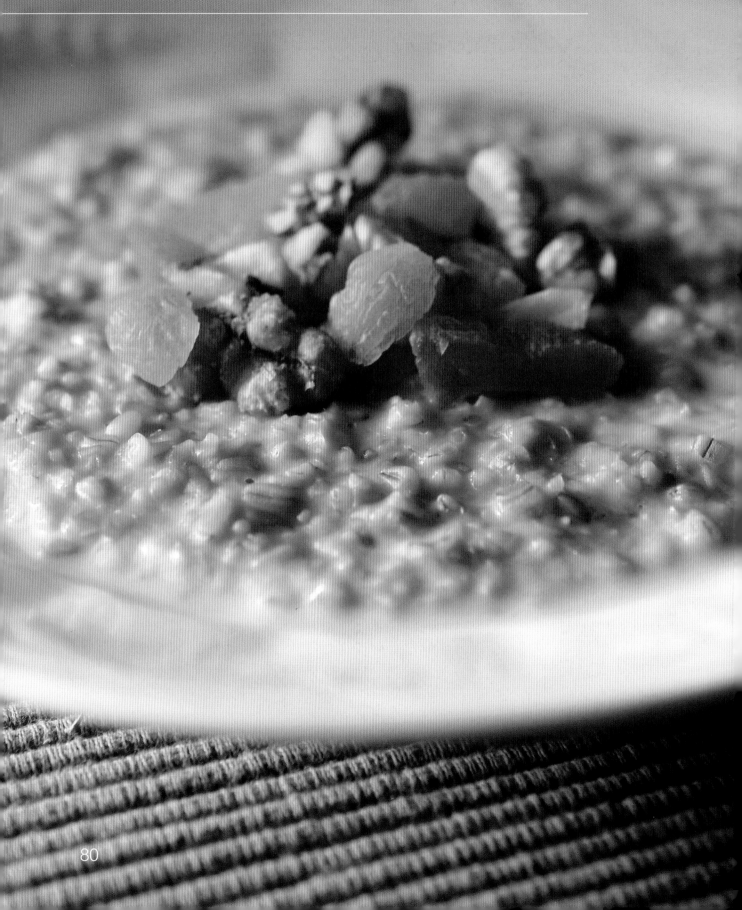

Steel-Cut Oats

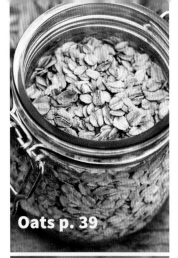

Oats p. 39

INGREDIENTS

- 1 cup steel-cut oats
- 4 cups unsweetened soy milk
- ¼ teaspoon salt
- 2 tablespoons honey
- Fresh or dried fruit and nuts for topping (optional)

INSTRUCTIONS

1. Soak steel-cut oats in water for a few hours or overnight. Discard soaking water and rinse well.

2. Place oats in a saucepan with soy milk, salt, and honey and mix well. Bring mixture to a boil, reduce to a simmer, and simmer for 35 to 45 minutes, stirring occasionally. For thinner oats, add additional soy milk or water.

Serve topped with fresh or dried fruits and nuts. Makes 4 servings.

Tip!

SERVING SIZE	TOTAL FAT	CHOLESTEROL	TOTAL CARBS	SUGARS
• 301 g	• 5.6 g	• 0 mg	• 38.5 g	• 11 g
CALORIES	SATURATED FAT	SODIUM	DIETARY FIBER	PROTEIN
• 252	• 0.8 g	• 190 mg	• 5.1 g	• 11.3 g

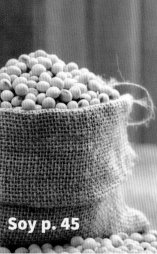

Soy p. 45

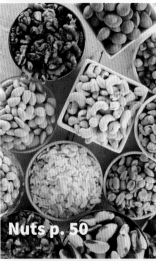

Nuts p. 50

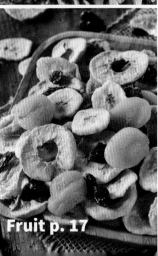

Fruit p. 17

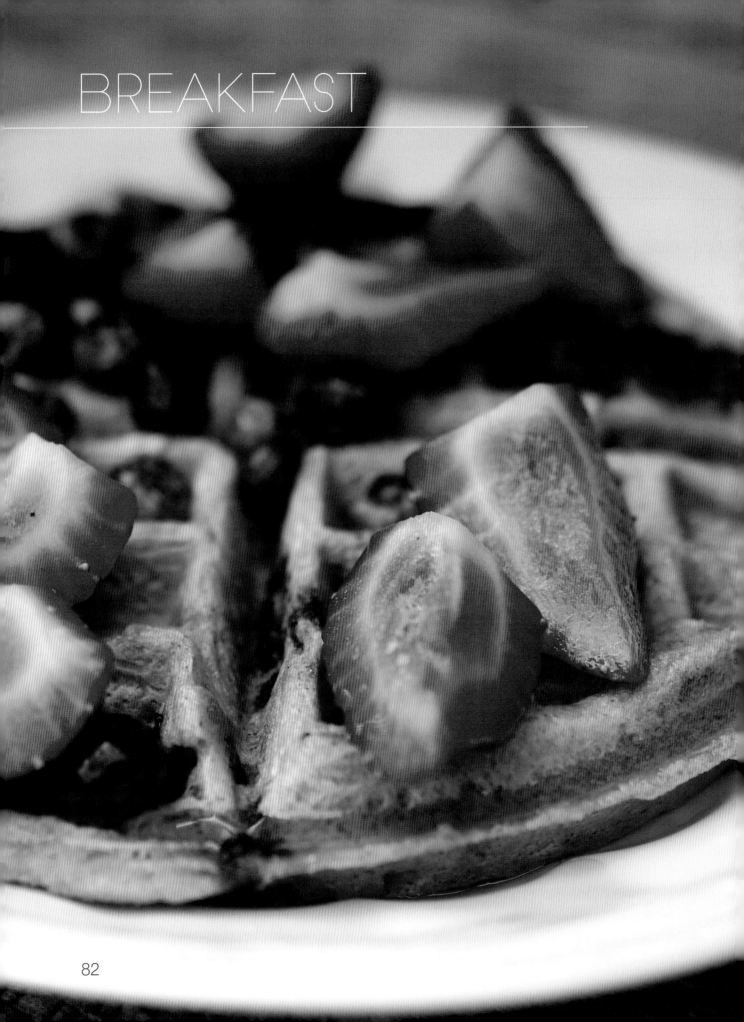

Berry Waffles

INGREDIENTS

- 2 cups rolled oats
- 1 cup whole-wheat flour
- ¼ cup ground flaxseed
- 4 cups unsweetened soy milk
- 5 pitted dates
- ¼ teaspoon salt
- 1 cup fresh or frozen berries of choice

INSTRUCTIONS

1. Combine oats, flour, soy milk, dates, and salt in a blender and blend until smooth. Allow mixture to sit for about 10 minutes to thicken, then mix in berries. Heat waffle iron and spray with nonstick cooking spray.

2. Pour waffle mixture into iron and cook according to manufacturer's instructions. Makes 5 Belgian-style waffles.

 Tip! Waffles may be frozen for later use. To freeze, cool waffles completely, then place in a freezer-safe bag or container. Waffles may be toasted in a toaster or toaster oven straight out of the freezer.

SERVING SIZE	TOTAL FAT	CHOLESTEROL	TOTAL CARBS	SUGARS
300 g	7.0 g	0 mg	54.1 g	10.2 g
CALORIES	SATURATED FAT	SODIUM	DIETARY FIBER	PROTEIN
333	1.3 g	154 mg	10.0 g	13.9 g

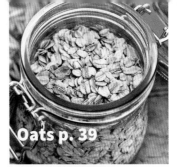
Oats p. 39

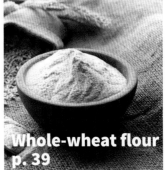
Whole-wheat flour p. 39

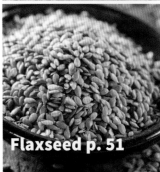
Flaxseed p. 51

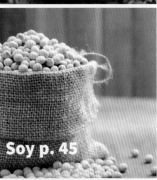
Soy p. 45

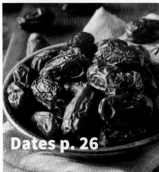
Dates p. 26

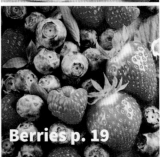
Berries p. 19

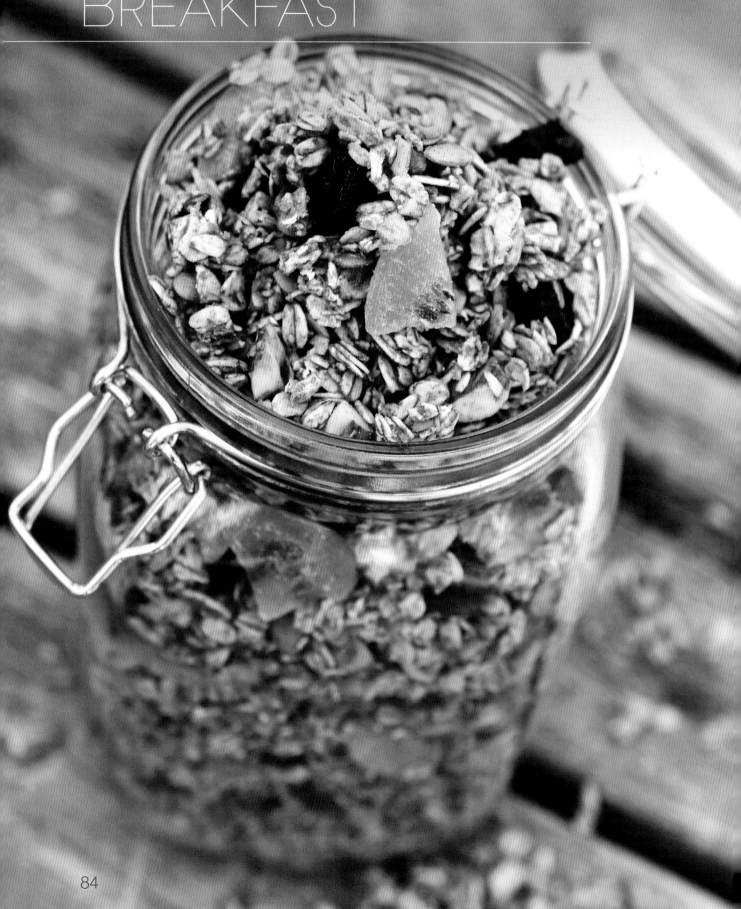

Granola

INGREDIENTS

- 1 cup raw cashews
- 2 cups pitted dates
- 1 cup water
- 1 cup honey
- 1 teaspoon salt
- 14 cups rolled oats
- 1 cup raw shelled sunflower seeds
- 1 cup raw shelled pumpkin seeds
- 1 cup raw whole almonds, roughly chopped
- 2 cups raw walnuts, roughly chopped

INSTRUCTIONS

1. Soak cashews in water for a couple of hours or overnight. Discard soaking water, then rinse and drain cashews. Place cashews, along with dates, water, honey, and salt, in a blender and blend until smooth.

2. Preheat oven to 180 degrees Fahrenheit. Combine the oats, sunflower seeds, pumpkin seeds, almonds, and walnuts in a large bowl and mix together, then add blended mixture. Mix well. Spread granola mixture in an even, single layer on several baking trays and bake in oven for 8 to 10 hours or until mixture is completely dry and crunchy. Stir and evenly spread granola mixture every 2 to 3 hours to ensure even cooking. Cool granola completely and store in an airtight container.

Tip! Recipe can be easily halved or even doubled as needed

SERVING SIZE	TOTAL FAT	CHOLESTEROL	TOTAL CARBS	SUGARS
56 g (½ cup)	8.9 g	0 mg	28.4 g	10.9 g
CALORIES	SATURATED FAT	SODIUM	DIETARY FIBER	PROTEIN
206	1.1 g	48 mg	3.8 g	5.5 g

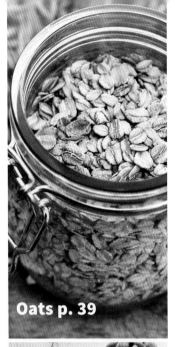

Oats p. 39

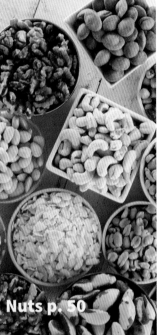

Nuts p. 50

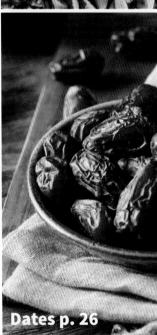

Dates p. 26

Cancer-Fighting Ingredients

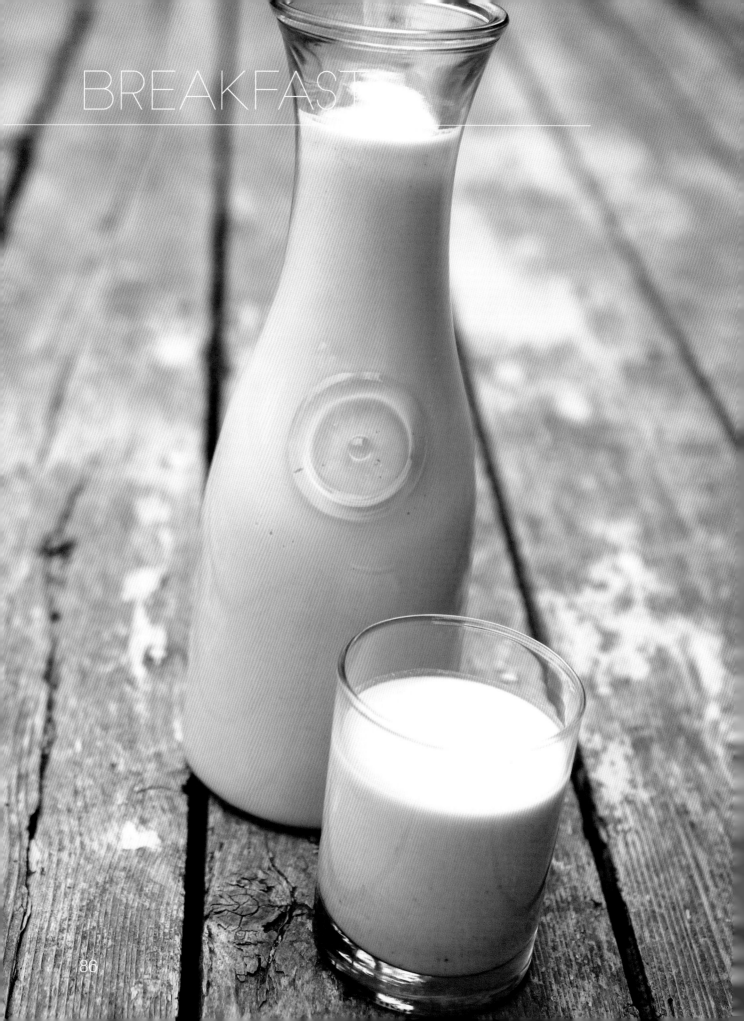

BREAKFAST

Nut Milk

INGREDIENTS

- 1 cup raw walnuts (or other raw nut of choice)
- 4 ½ to 5 cups water, divided
- ¼ teaspoon salt (optional)
- 1 to 2 tablespoons honey or maple syrup or 3 to 4 dates (optional)

INSTRUCTIONS

1. Soak walnuts for 8 hours or overnight. Rinse well, drain, and add walnuts to blender with 1 cup fresh water.

2. If adding salt and sweetener, add them here. Blend until very smooth, then add remaining 3 ½ to 4 cups fresh water, depending on how thick you like your milk. Blend well. If you find the milk a little gritty, you may strain it through a cheesecloth or a nut-milk bag. Makes 5 servings.

If you strain your milk, save the pulp to add to other recipes like breads and muffins. Also, if you wish to add sweetener, add it to the milk after you have strained it.

Tip! Use this recipe to make seed milk by swapping nuts for seeds (try sunflower or pumpkin).

SERVING SIZE	TOTAL FAT	CHOLESTEROL	TOTAL CARBS	SUGARS
• 261 g	• 16.0 g	• 0 mg	• 2.4 g	• 0 g
CALORIES	SATURATED FAT	SODIUM	DIETARY FIBER	PROTEIN
• 168	• 1.2 g	• 7 mg	• 2.4 g	• 4 g

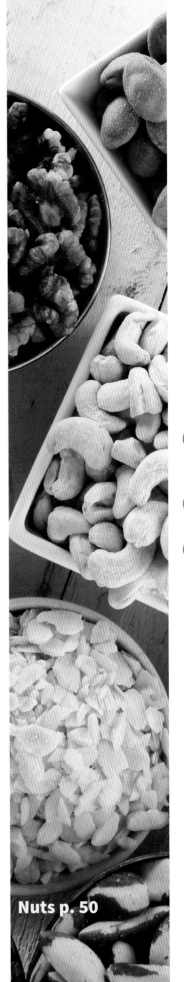

Nuts p. 50

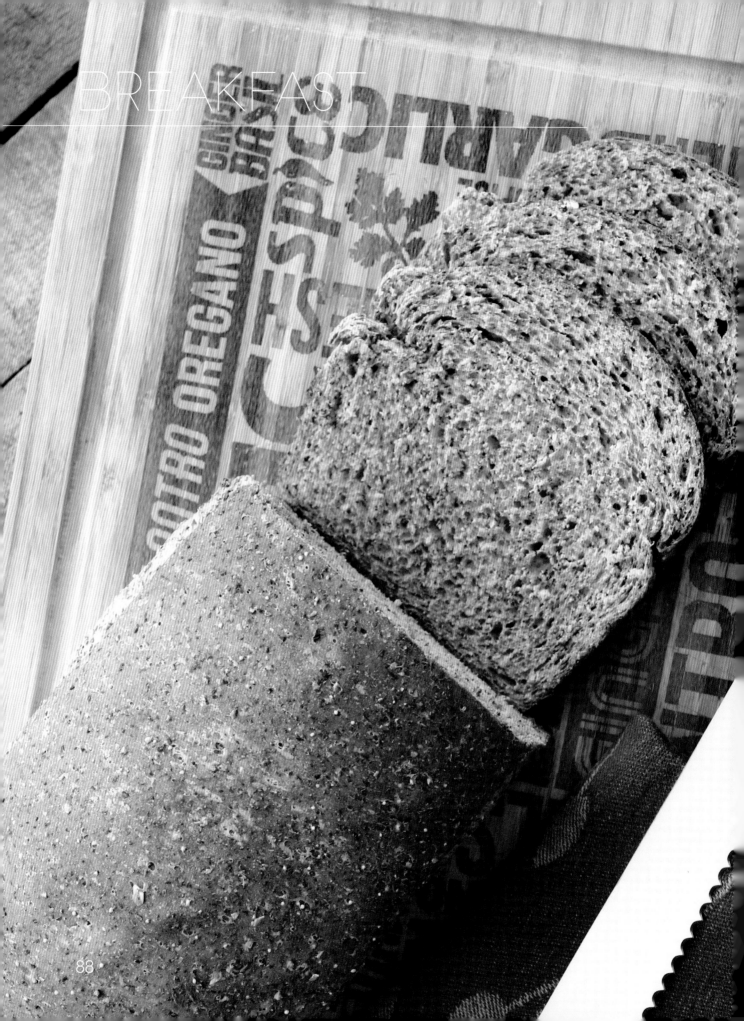

Multigrain Flax Bread

INGREDIENTS

- 3 cups all-purpose flour
- 1 ½ cups whole-wheat flour
- 1 cup 12-grain flour (or other multigrain flour)
- 1 cup ground flaxseeds
- ½ cup 12 grain cereal (or other multigrain cereal)
- 3 tablespoons gluten flour
- 3 tablespoons soy milk powder
- 1 ½ teaspoons salt
- 3 cups warm water
- 3 teaspoons instant yeast
- 3 tablespoons oil
- ¼ cup honey

INSTRUCTIONS

1. Mix dry ingredients in a large bowl. In a smaller bowl, mix together wet ingredients, then pour into dry. Knead dough by hand for 7 to 10 minutes, or knead in batches in a food processor using the dough blade 1 minute per batch (the number of batches will depend on the size of your food processor). Alternatively, use your bread maker to make this recipe. Spray 2 medium loaf pans with nonstick cooking spray.

2. Divide dough into 2 equal pieces, shape into loaves, and place loaves in pans. Let rise 30 to 40 minutes, then bake at 350 degrees Fahrenheit for 30 to 35 minutes or until bread is golden brown on top and sounds hollow when tapped at the bottom. Allow bread to cool completely before eating. Makes 2 loaves and 12 slices per loaf.

 Store bread for a day or two before eating to fully develop flavor and optimum nutritional benefit.

 Tip! Recipe can be easily halved or doubled as needed. Note, too, that bread freezes well.

To save time in the future, combine all the dry ingredients except yeast and salt to make your own "instant" multigrain bread flour. When you want to make the bread, simply use about 6 ½ cups of the flour (for 2 loaves) and add the remaining ingredients.

SERVING SIZE	TOTAL FAT	CHOLESTEROL	TOTAL CARBS	SUGARS
• 148 g (2 slices)	• 8.2 g	• 0 mg	• 65.1 g	• 7.7 g
CALORIES	SATURATED FAT	SODIUM	DIETARY FIBER	PROTEIN
• 391	• 1.1 g	• 304 mg	• 10.1 g	• 14.1 g

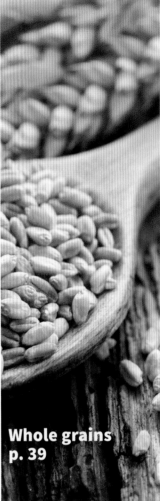

Whole grains p. 39

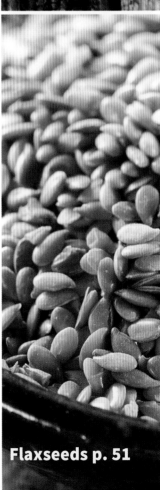

Flaxseeds p. 51

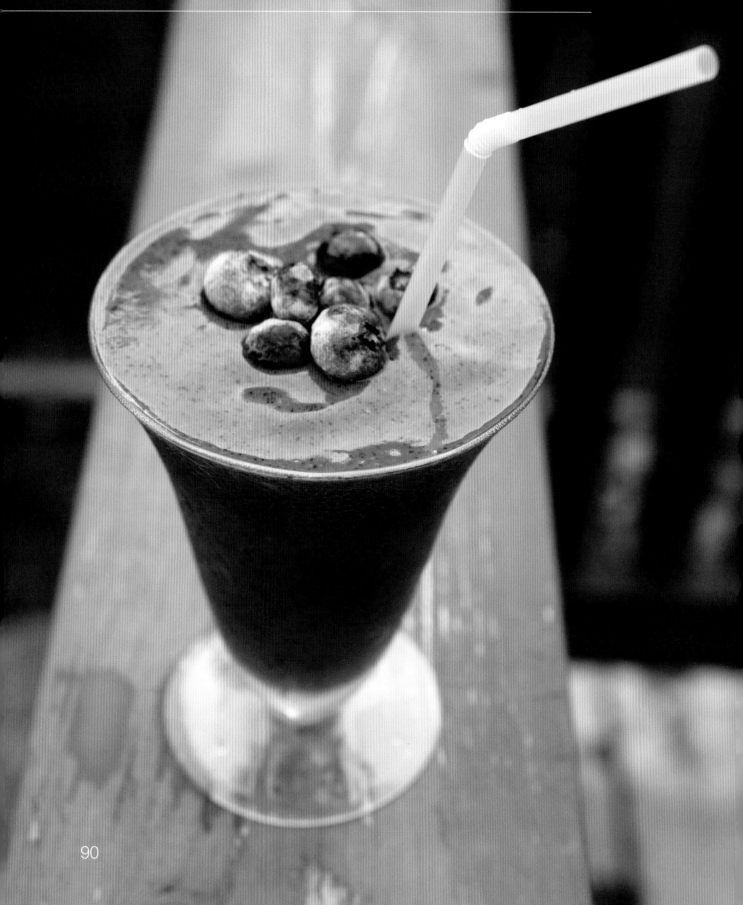

Very Berry Smoothie

INGREDIENTS

- 1 banana
- ½ cup unsweetened soy milk
- 1 cup frozen berries

INSTRUCTIONS

1. Dice up banana and freeze for at least 2 hours or overnight. Add soy milk and frozen banana to a blender and blend.

2. Add frozen berries to the soy-banana mixture and blend until smooth. Depending on your blender, you may need to add the berries a few at a time to ensure the fruit blends smoothly. If you still have trouble, add a little more soy milk to help the process along. Makes 1 serving.

Tip! Remember that the recipe can be doubled, tripled, even quadrupled as needed.

SERVING SIZE	TOTAL FAT	CHOLESTEROL	TOTAL CARBS	SUGARS
• 388 g	• 2.4 g	• 0 mg	• 49.5 g	• 29.8 g
CALORIES	**SATURATED FAT**	**SODIUM**	**DIETARY FIBER**	**PROTEIN**
• 223	• 0.5 g	• 22 mg	• 7.1 g	• 5.4 g

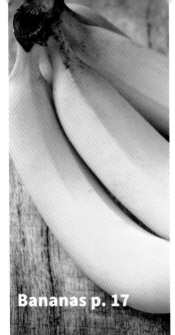

Bananas p. 17

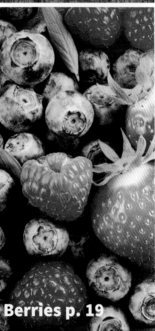

Berries p. 19

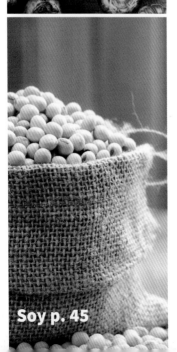

Soy p. 45

BREAKFAST

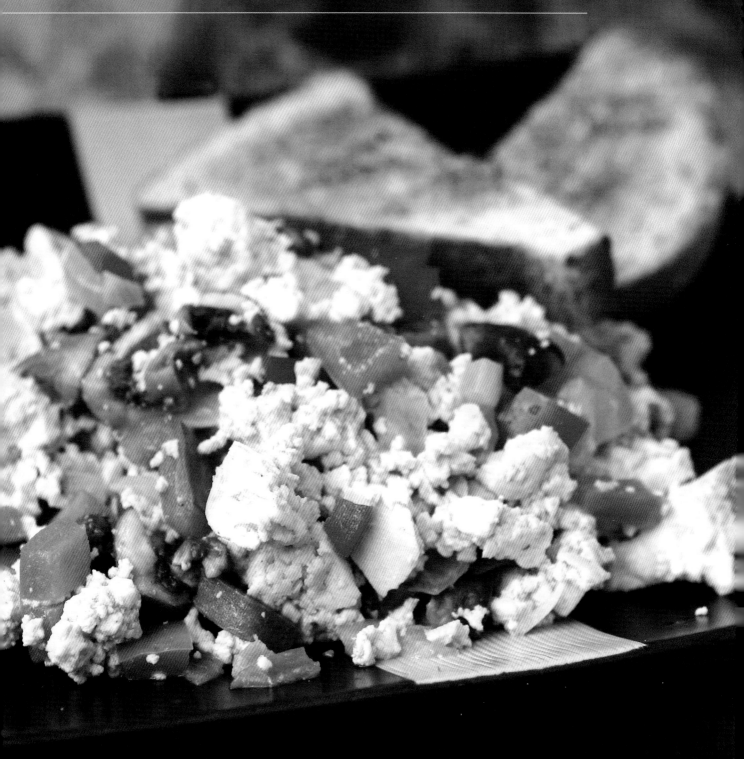

Tofu Veggie Scramble

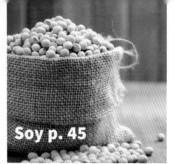
Soy p. 45

INGREDIENTS

- 1 cup chopped onion
- 2 tablespoons olive oil
- 2 cloves garlic, minced
- 1 cup white button or cremini mushrooms, sliced
- ½ red bell pepper, chopped
- 1 medium carrot, chopped
- 1 package extra-firm tofu
- ¼ teaspoon turmeric
- ½ teaspoon salt
- 1 cup fresh baby spinach

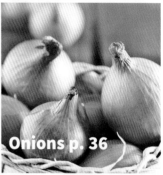
Onions p. 36

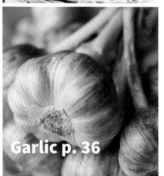
Garlic p. 36

INSTRUCTIONS

1. In a large pan, sauté onion in oil until softened, about 5 minutes. Add minced garlic and sauté another minute, then add mushrooms, bell pepper, and carrot and sauté for 5 to 7 minutes or until veggies have softened but still have some bite.

2. Crumble tofu and add to veggie mixture, then sprinkle on turmeric and salt and stir until evenly mixed and tofu is heated through. Add spinach and stir until just wilted. Makes 6 servings (approximately ½ cup per serving).

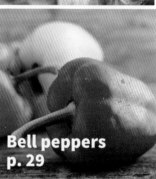
Bell peppers p. 29

SERVING SIZE	TOTAL FAT	CHOLESTEROL	TOTAL CARBS	SUGARS
120 g	10.1 g	0 mg	5.8 g	2.0 g
CALORIES	SATURATED FAT	SODIUM	DIETARY FIBER	PROTEIN
148	1.7 g	217 mg	1.1 g	9.6 g

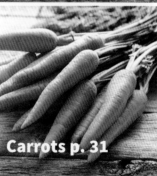
Carrots p. 31

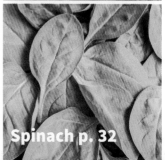
Spinach p. 32

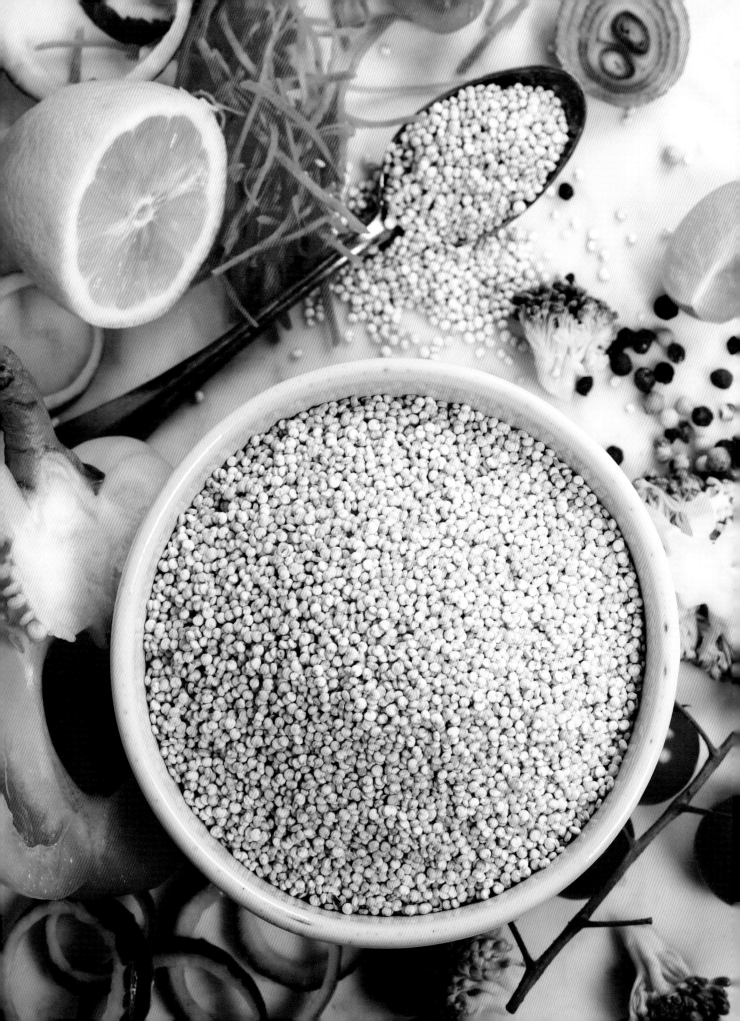

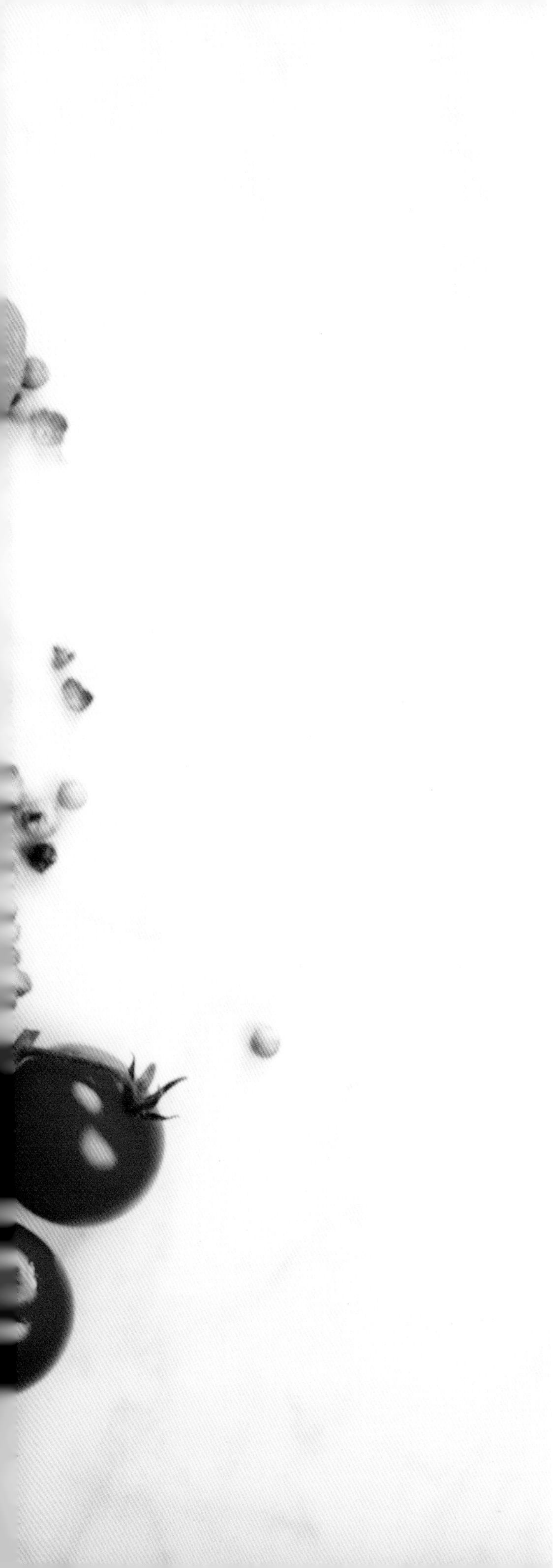

Mains

Black Bean Burgers

Spinach-Basil Pesto

Lentil Stew

Black-Eyed Bean Stew

Tofu Salad

Vegan Mac and Cheese

Broccoli "Cheese" Potatoes

Sweet Potato Burritos

Creamy Rice 'n' Sprouts

Hummus

Tomato Soup

Veggie Wrap With "Cream Cheese"

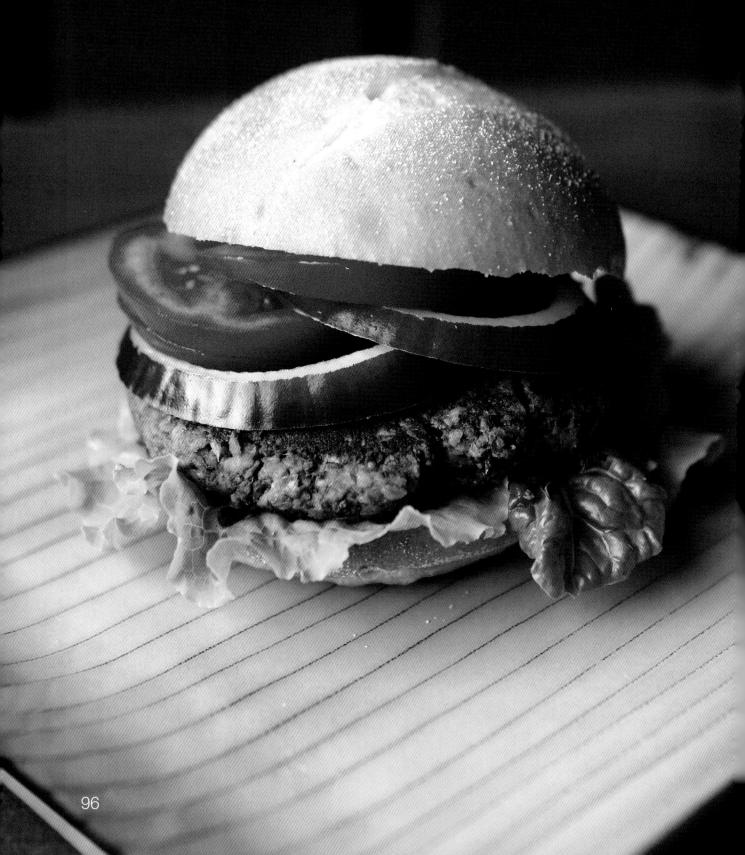

Black Bean Burgers

INGREDIENTS

- 1 (19-oz) can black beans, drained and rinsed (or 2 cups cooked black beans)
- 1 cup diced cremini mushrooms
- 1 tablespoon olive oil
- ½ cup finely diced onions
- 2 cloves garlic, minced
- ⅔ cup raw walnuts, finely chopped
- ¾ cup quick oats
- ½ teaspoon salt (or to taste)

INSTRUCTIONS

1. Put beans in a large bowl and set aside. Sauté mushrooms in olive oil on medium to medium-high heat until they have browned and the water from the mushrooms has evaporated. Add onions and cook for 2 minutes, then add garlic and walnuts and cook for another 2 minutes. Mushroom mixture should be fairly dry. If still wet, cook for a little longer until more water has evaporated.

2. Add mushroom mixture to beans, then add quick oats and salt. Mash mixture with a fork or your hands until it is well mixed and comes together. Alternatively, place all ingredients in a food processor and process for a few seconds, just until the mixture is evenly mixed. Scoop out ½-cup portions of the mixture and form into patties.

3. To bake patties, preheat oven to 375 degrees Fahrenheit, then lightly spray a baking sheet with nonstick cooking spray. Place patties on baking sheet and bake for 7 to 10 minutes on each side or until golden brown and warmed through. To cook patties on stovetop, lightly spray a nonstick skillet with nonstick cooking spray and cook patties over medium heat on each side for 3 to 5 minutes or until each side is lightly browned and the patties are heated through.

4. Serve on whole-wheat buns with lettuce, tomato, onion, and any other favorite toppings. Makes 5 patties.

Tip! Patties freeze well. Double the recipe and freeze uncooked patties for later use.

SERVING SIZE	TOTAL FAT	CHOLESTEROL	TOTAL CARBS	SUGARS
156 g (1 pattie)	15.1 g	0 mg	26.3 g	0.9 g
CALORIES	SATURATED FAT	SODIUM	DIETARY FIBER	PROTEIN
281	1.3 g	247 mg	8.0 g	10.5 g

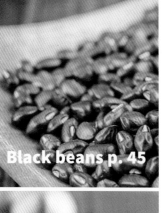

Black beans p. 45

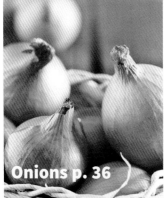

Onions p. 36

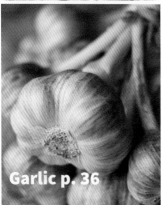

Garlic p. 36

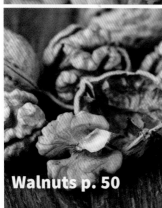

Walnuts p. 50

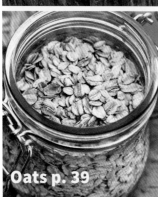

Oats p. 39

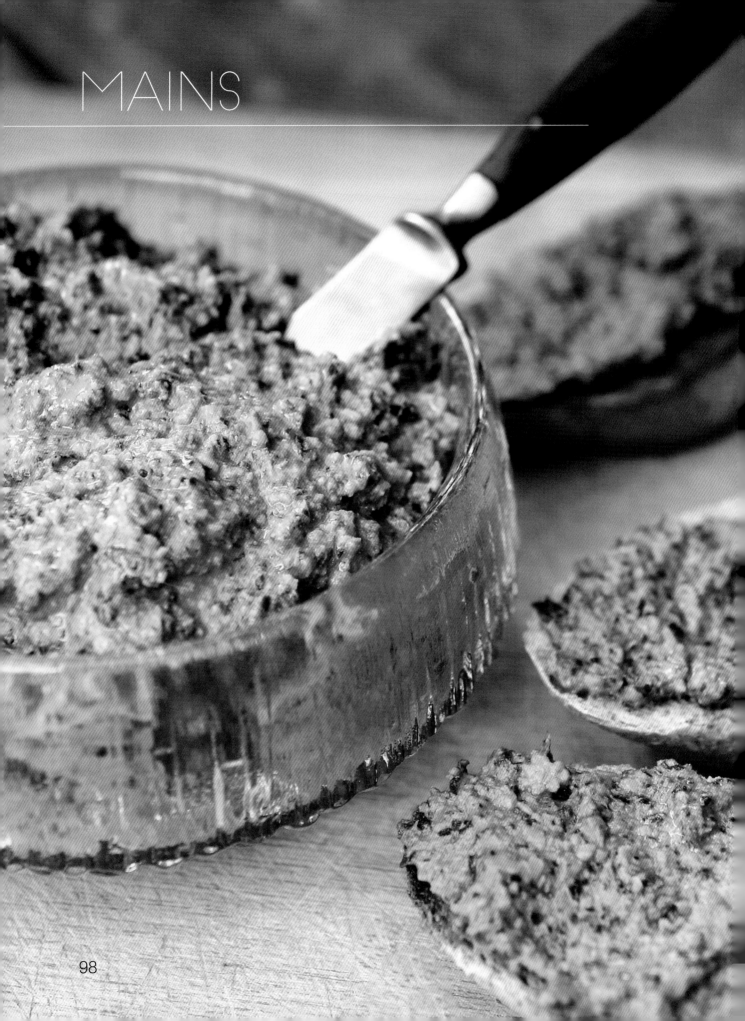

Spinach-Basil Pesto

INGREDIENTS

- 1 packed cup spinach
- 1 packed cup fresh basil
- 1 cup raw walnuts
- ⅓ cup extra-virgin olive oil
- 2 cloves garlic
- ¼ teaspoon salt

INSTRUCTIONS

1. Blend spinach, basil, walnuts, oil, garlic, and salt in a food processor until everything is evenly combined but there is some texture remaining.

2. Add 2 tablespoons pesto to a single serving of whole-wheat pasta for a delicious pasta dish, or spread pesto on whole-wheat bread for a quick meal. Add sautéed vegetables to bread and pesto for a hearty sandwich. Makes 10 servings (approximately 2 tablespoons per serving).

Tip! Pesto freezes well. Divide into 2-tablespoon portions and freeze in small containers or in an ice tray.

SERVING SIZE	TOTAL FAT	CHOLESTEROL	TOTAL CARBS	SUGARS
• 32 g (2 tbsp)	• 15.5 g	• 0 mg	• 1.8 g	• NA
CALORIES	SATURATED FAT	SODIUM	DIETARY FIBER	PROTEIN
• 152	• 1.7 g	• 64 mg	• 1.4 g	• 2.4 g

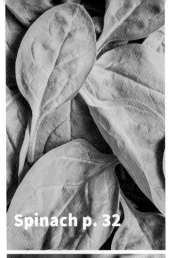
Spinach p. 32

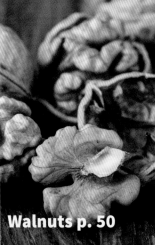
Walnuts p. 50

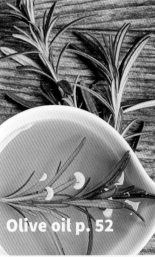
Olive oil p. 52

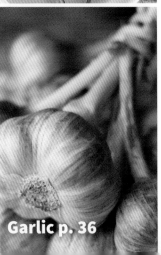
Garlic p. 36

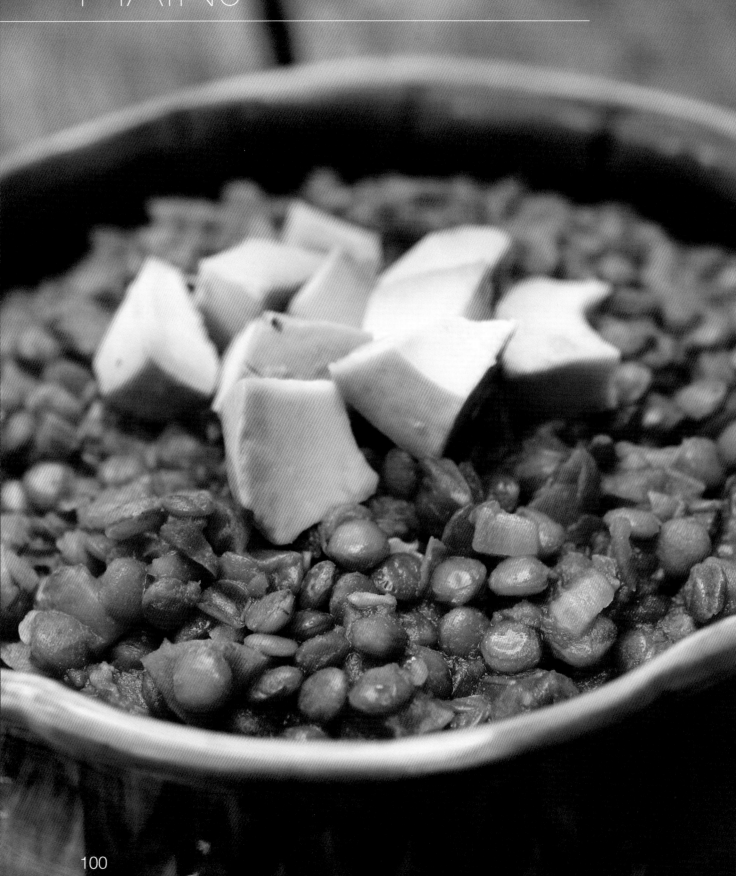

Lentil Stew

INGREDIENTS

- 1 cup chopped onions
- 1 stalk celery, diced
- 2 tablespoons olive oil
- 2 cloves garlic, minced
- ½ cup diced tomatoes
- 1 dried bay leaf
- 3 cups water
- 1 cup dry green lentils
- 1 carrot, diced
- ½ teaspoon salt

INSTRUCTIONS

1. In a medium saucepan, sauté onions and celery in olive oil for about 5 minutes. Add garlic and sauté another minute. Next, add diced tomatoes, bay leaf, water, and lentils. Bring mixture to a boil, reduce to a simmer, and simmer for 25 minutes.

2. Add carrot and simmer another 15 minutes, or until lentils and carrots are tender. Add salt and taste for seasonings, adjusting as necessary. For a thinner soup, add a little more water. Top stew with avocado if desired. Makes 5 servings (approximately 1 cup per serving).

SERVING SIZE	TOTAL FAT	CHOLESTEROL	TOTAL CARBS	SUGARS
• 260 g	• 6.0 g	• 0 mg	• 21.6 g	• 2.5 g
CALORIES	SATURATED FAT	SODIUM	DIETARY FIBER	PROTEIN
• 164	• 0.9 g	• 252 mg	• 8.0 g	• 6.8 g

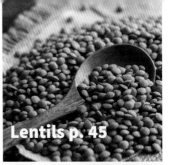

Lentils p. 45

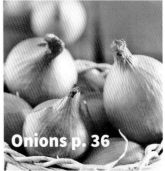

Onions p. 36

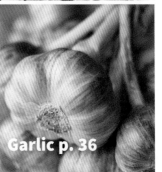

Garlic p. 36

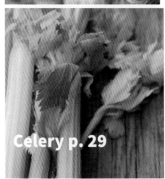

Celery p. 29

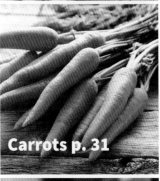

Carrots p. 31

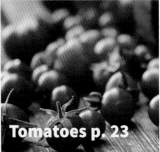

Tomatoes p. 23

Cancer-Fighting Ingredients

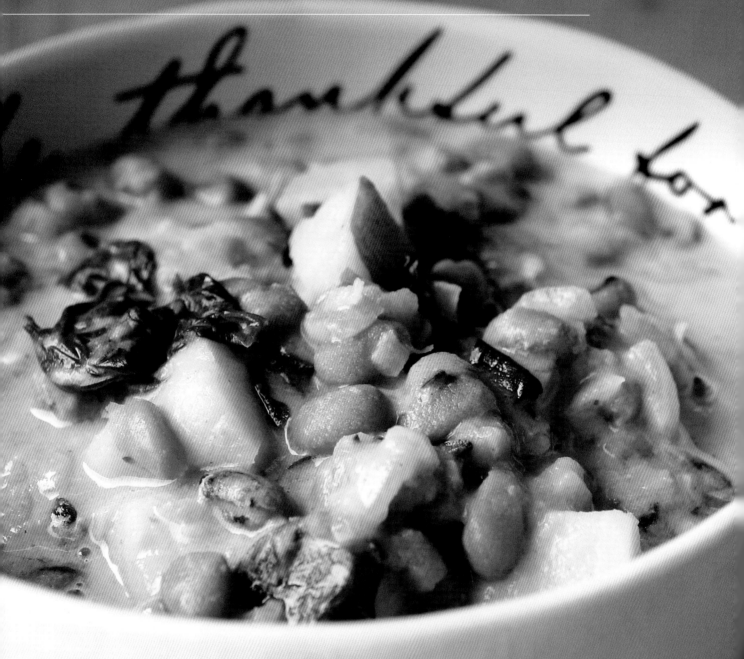

Black-Eyed Peas Stew

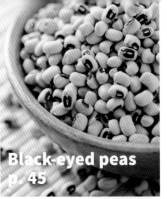

Black-eyed peas
p. 45

INGREDIENTS

- 1 cup chopped onions
- 2 tablespoons olive oil
- 2 cloves garlic
- ¼ teaspoon turmeric
- 1 ½ cups water
- ½ cup coconut milk
- 2 medium red potatoes, unpeeled and diced into bite-sized pieces
- 1 (19oz) can black-eyed peas, drained and rinsed (or 2 cups of cooked black-eyed peas)
- 1 ½ cups chopped kale
- ¾ teaspoon salt

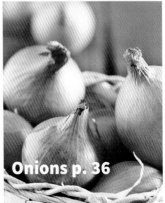

Onions p. 36

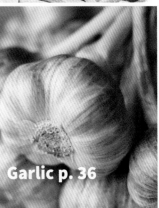

Garlic p. 36

INSTRUCTIONS

1. In a medium saucepan, sauté onions in olive oil for 5 to 7 minutes, then add garlic and sauté another minute. Add turmeric and stir to combine, then add water, coconut milk, and potatoes. Bring mixture to a boil, reduce to a simmer, and simmer for 10 to 15 minutes, or until potatoes are tender.

2. Add black-eyed peas and cook 3 to 5 minutes, until beans are warmed through. Add kale, stir, and cook for 2 to 3 minutes, or until kale is just wilted. Add salt, stir to combine, and taste for seasonings, adjusting as necessary. If you want a thinner stew, just add a little more water. Makes 6 servings (approximately 1 cup per serving).

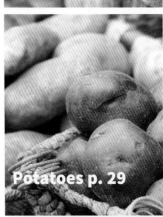

Potatoes p. 29

SERVING SIZE	TOTAL FAT	CHOLESTEROL	TOTAL CARBS	SUGARS
269 g	7 g	0 mg	26.2 g	1.7 g
CALORIES	SATURATED FAT	SODIUM	DIETARY FIBER	PROTEIN
182	2.1 g	323 mg	4.6 g	6.3 g

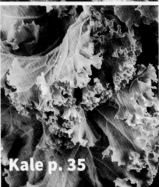

Kale p. 35

Cancer-Fighting Ingredients

MAINS

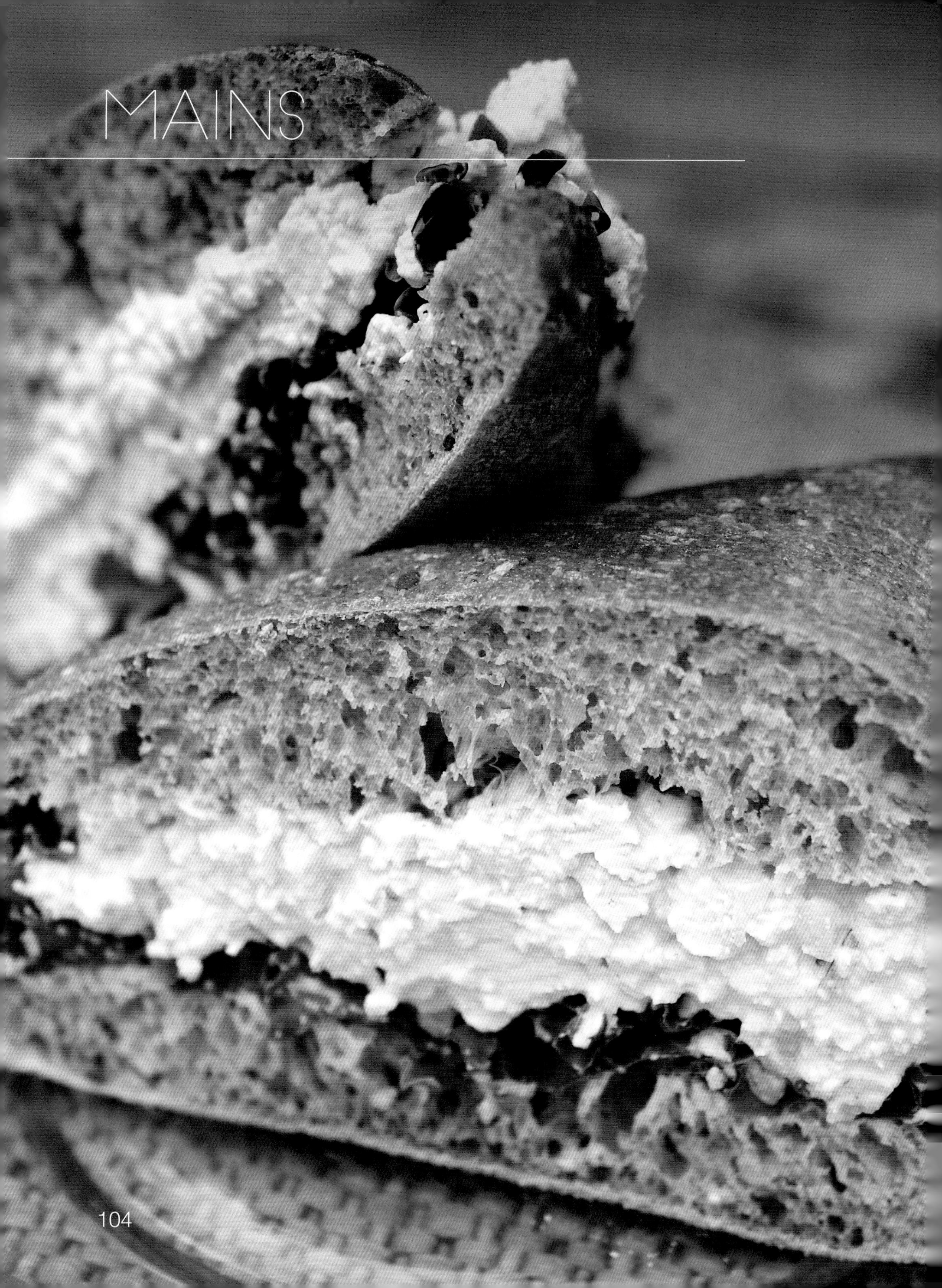

Tofu Salad

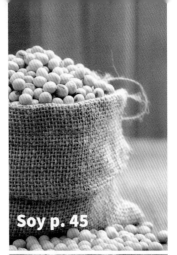

Soy p. 45

INGREDIENTS

- 1 package extra-firm tofu
- ¾ cup finely diced celery
- ¼ cup finely diced red onion
- 1 to 2 cloves garlic, minced
- ⅓ cup avocado oil (or other light-tasting oil)
- ½ cup unsweetened soy milk
- 1 tablespoon honey
- ½ teaspoon turmeric
- ¾ teaspoon salt

INSTRUCTIONS

1. Crumble tofu into a large bowl, squeezing out any excess liquid. To this bowl, add celery, onion, and garlic and mix to combine.

2. In a blender, blend oil, soy milk, honey, turmeric, and salt until well combined. Pour blended mixture into tofu mixture, and mix until everything is evenly combined. Chill in the refrigerator until ready to use. Makes 6 servings (approximately ½ cup per serving).

SERVING SIZE	TOTAL FAT	CHOLESTEROL	TOTAL CARBS	SUGARS
• 119 g	• 18 g	• 0 mg	• 5.9 g	• 3.4 g
CALORIES	SATURATED FAT	SODIUM	DIETARY FIBER	PROTEIN
• 234	• 3 g	• 316 mg	• NA	• 10.3 g

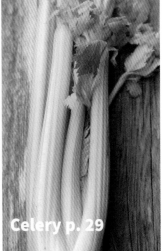

Celery p. 29

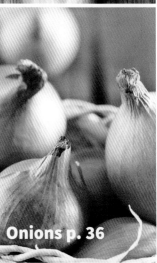

Onions p. 36

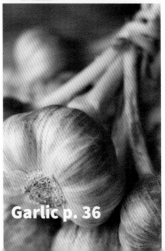

Garlic p. 36

Cancer-Fighting Ingredients

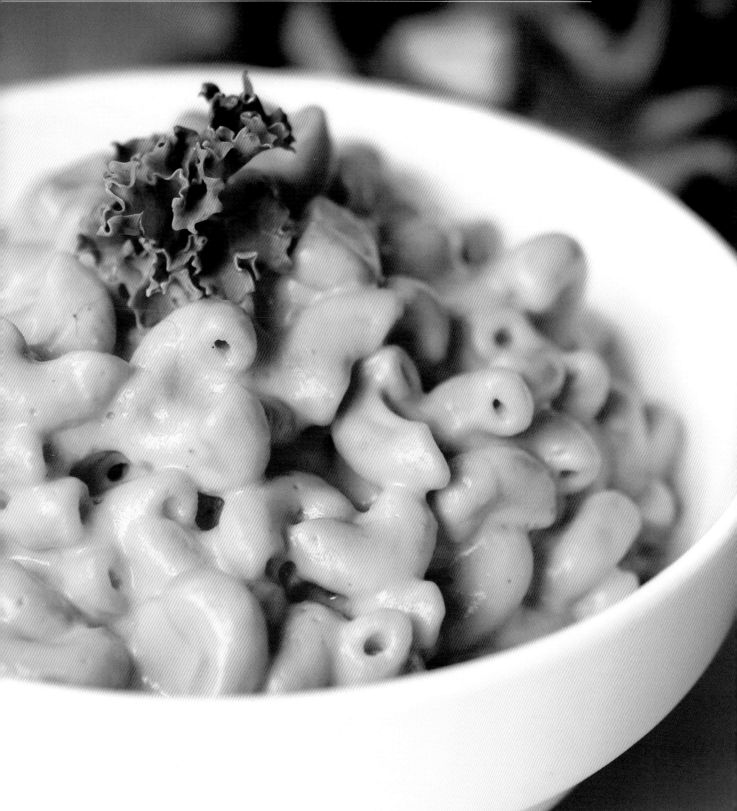

Vegan Mac and Cheese

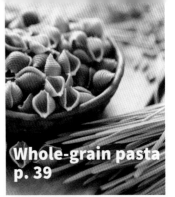

Whole-grain pasta p. 39

INGREDIENTS

- 1 cup chopped onions
- 2 cloves garlic
- 2 tablespoons olive oil
- ⅔ cup raw cashews, soaked
- 2 cups water
- ¼ cup roasted red bell peppers
- 1 teaspoon salt
- 1 package whole-wheat elbow macaroni (or other whole-wheat pasta)

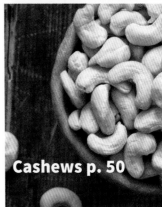

Cashews p. 50

INSTRUCTIONS

1. Sauté onions and garlic in olive oil until softened. In a blender, combine the cooked onion and garlic mixture with the cashews, water, bell peppers, and salt and blend until very smooth. Cook "cheese" mixture on stove over medium heat for 10 minutes, stirring constantly. Sauce will thicken as it cooks.

2. Cook macaroni in lightly salted water until al dente (cooked but with some bite). Drain, add "cheese" sauce, and stir to combine. Let sit for 5 to 10 minutes as pasta absorbs sauce and thickens. Stir once more to mix. Makes 6 servings (approximately 1 cup per serving).

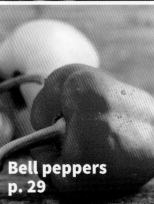

Bell peppers p. 29

SERVING SIZE	TOTAL FAT	CHOLESTEROL	TOTAL CARBS	SUGARS
• 195 g	• 11.6 g	• 0 mg	• 51.7 g	• 4.3 g
CALORIES	SATURATED FAT	SODIUM	DIETARY FIBER	PROTEIN
• 327	• 1.6 g	• 440 mg	• 7.5 g	• 10.2 g

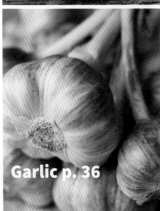

Garlic p. 36

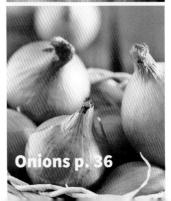

Onions p. 36

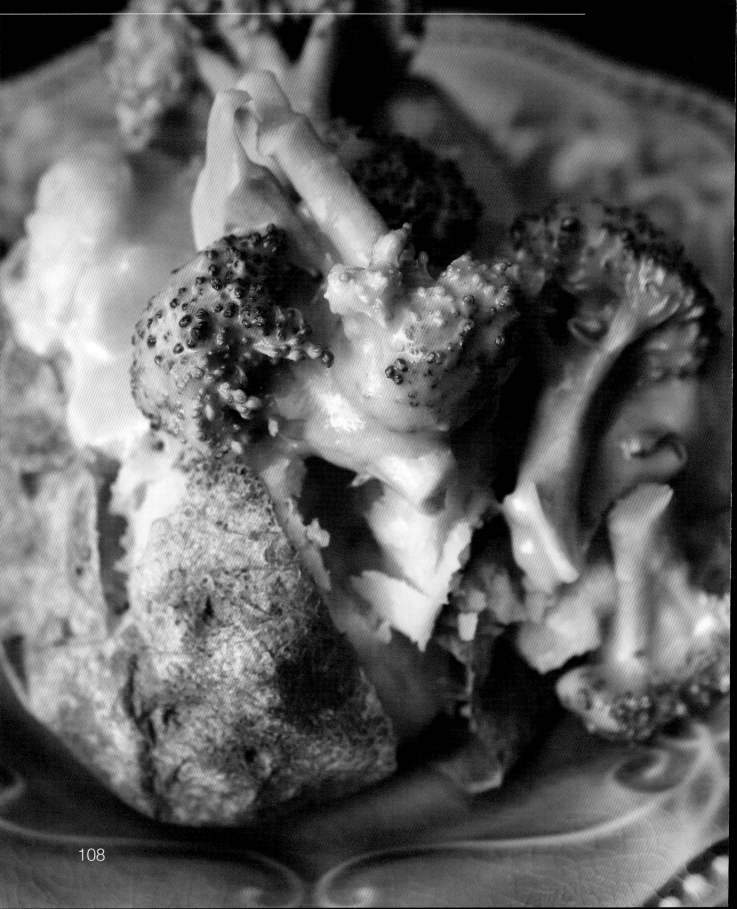

Broccoli "Cheese" Potatoes

INGREDIENTS

- 4 medium baking potatoes
- 1 cup chopped onions
- 2 cloves garlic
- 2 tablespoons extra-virgin olive oil
- $\frac{2}{3}$ cup raw cashews, soaked
- 2 cups water
- $\frac{1}{4}$ cup roasted red bell peppers
- 1 teaspoon salt
- 3 cups diced broccoli

INSTRUCTIONS

1. Preheat oven to 425 degrees Fahrenheit. Wash and dry potatoes and prick them all over with a fork. Place potatoes on a baking sheet or directly on the oven rack and bake for 45 to 60 minutes, or until tender. Alternatively, microwave potatoes on high for 7 to 10 minutes, or until tender.

2. Meanwhile, sauté onions and garlic in olive oil until softened. In a blender, combine cooked onion and garlic mixture with the cashews, water, bell peppers, and salt and blend until very smooth. Cook "cheese" mixture on stove over medium heat for 5 minutes, stirring constantly. Add diced broccoli and cook for 5 to 7 minutes, or until broccoli is warmed through and softened but still has a bite. Pour broccoli and "cheese" sauce over each baked potato. Makes 4 servings.

SERVING SIZE	TOTAL FAT	CHOLESTEROL	TOTAL CARBS	SUGARS
440 g	16.2 g	0 mg	44.8 g	5.6 g
CALORIES	SATURATED FAT	SODIUM	DIETARY FIBER	PROTEIN
346	2.4 g	699 mg	5.4 g	9.2 g

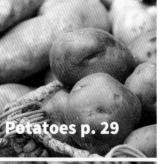
Potatoes p. 29

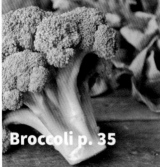
Broccoli p. 35

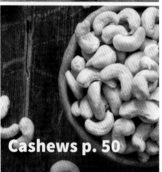
Cashews p. 50

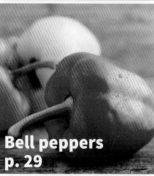
Bell peppers p. 29

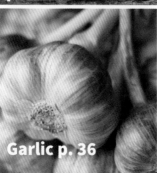
Garlic p. 36

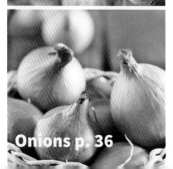
Onions p. 36

Cancer-Fighting Ingredients

MAINS

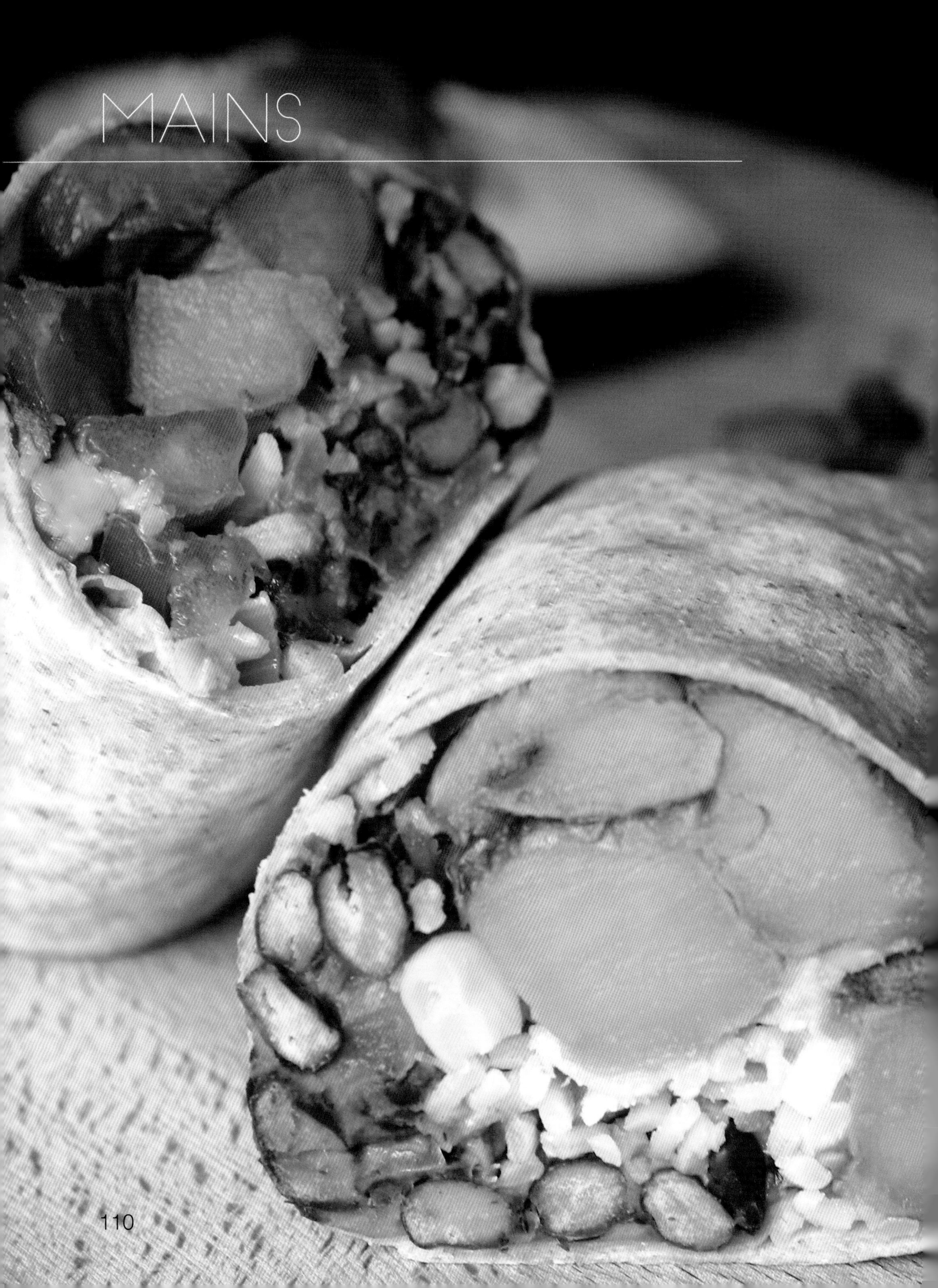

Sweet Potato Burritos

INGREDIENTS

- 2 medium sweet potatoes
- 1 tablespoon olive oil
- Salt (optional)
- 1 cup cooked black beans
- 4 whole-wheat tortillas
- 1 cup cooked brown rice
- ½ cup diced red onions
- ½ cup diced tomatoes
- ½ cup corn
- 1 avocado, diced

INSTRUCTIONS

1. Preheat oven to 400 degrees Fahrenheit. Wash potatoes well and cut them into bite-sized pieces. Toss potatoes in olive oil and spread in a single layer on a baking sheet. Bake potatoes for 25 to 30 minutes, or until potatoes are tender. Sprinkle on a little salt if desired.

2. Put about ¼ cup rice and ¼ cup beans (or as desired) on each tortilla, then sprinkle on onions, tomatoes, corn, and avocado. Makes 4 burritos.

SERVING SIZE	TOTAL FAT	CHOLESTEROL	TOTAL CARBS	SUGARS
297 g	15.3 g	0 mg	65 g	4.6 g
CALORIES	SATURATED FAT	SODIUM	DIETARY FIBER	PROTEIN
428	2.6 g	178 mg	13 g	11.9 g

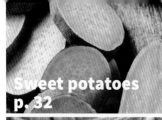
Sweet potatoes p. 32

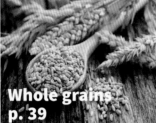
Whole grains p. 39

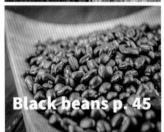
Black beans p. 45

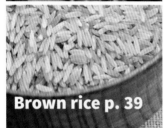
Brown rice p. 39

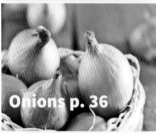
Onions p. 36

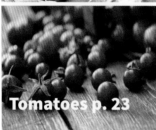
Tomatoes p. 23

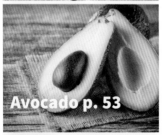
Avocado p. 53

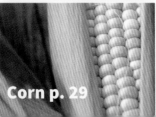
Corn p. 29

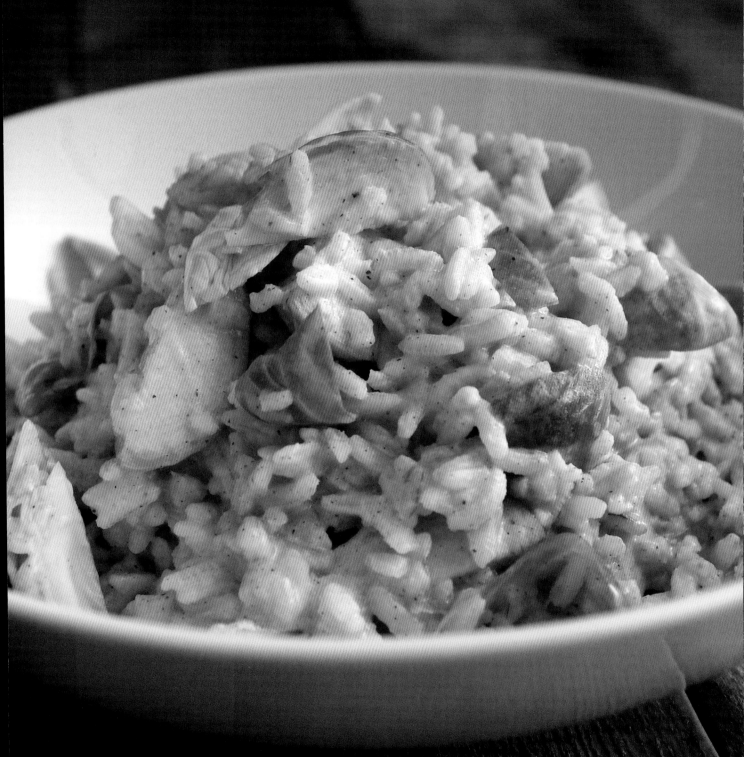

Creamy Rice 'n' Sprouts

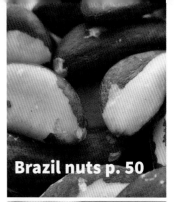
Brazil nuts p. 50

INGREDIENTS

- ½ cup chopped onions
- 1 tablespoon olive oil
- ½ cup raw Brazil nuts
- 2 cloves garlic
- 1 tablespoon cornstarch
- ¾ cup water
- ¼ teaspoon salt
- 1 ½ cups quartered or shredded Brussels sprouts
- 2 ½ cups cooked brown rice

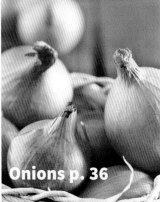
Onions p. 36

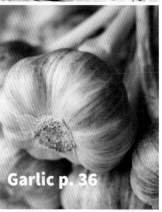
Garlic p. 36

INSTRUCTIONS

1. In a small saucepan, sauté onions in olive oil for 5 to 7 minutes, or until onions have softened. Put cooked onions in a blender along with Brazil nuts, garlic, cornstarch, water, and salt and blend until smooth.

2. Gently steam Brussels sprouts in a saucepan with a little water or in a steamer basket for 5 to 7 minutes, or until just tender. Add steamed Brussels sprouts, rice, and Brazil nut gravy to a pot and mix together. If mixture is a little dry, add a little water. Taste and add additional salt if necessary. Makes 4 servings (approximately 1 cup per serving).

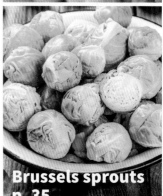
Brussels sprouts p. 35

SERVING SIZE	TOTAL FAT	CHOLESTEROL	TOTAL CARBS	SUGARS
152 g	15.5 g	0 mg	35.9 g	1.9 g
CALORIES	SATURATED FAT	SODIUM	DIETARY FIBER	PROTEIN
293	3.2 g	158 mg	4.4 g	7 g

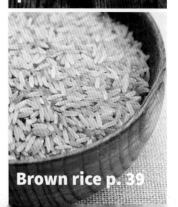
Brown rice p. 39

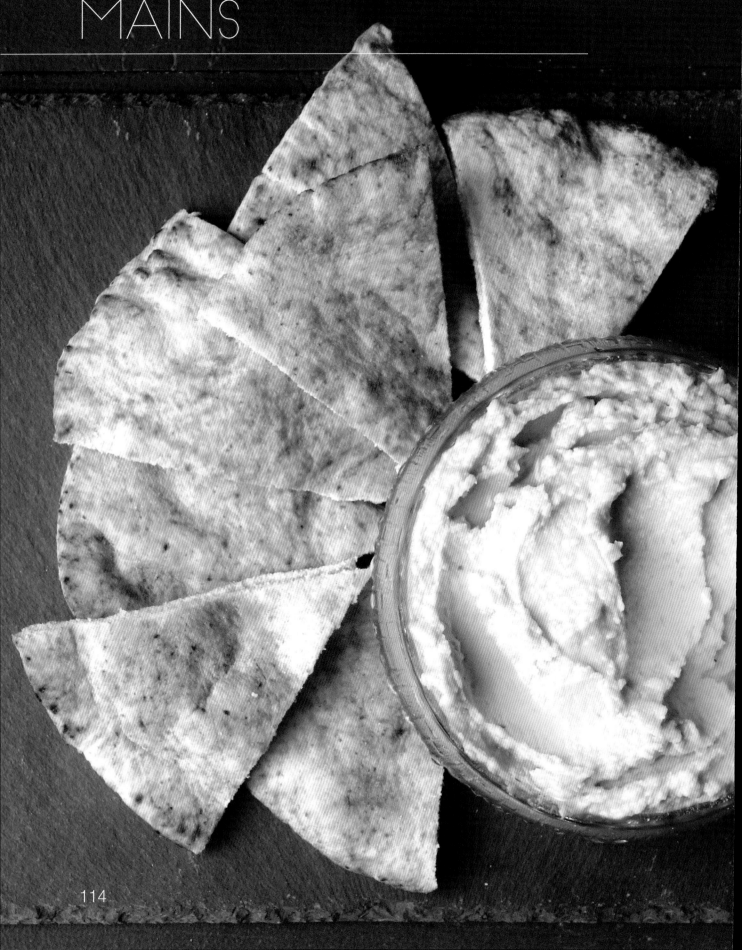

Hummus

INGREDIENTS

- 1 (19-oz) can chickpeas (or 2 cups cooked chickpeas)
- 2 cloves garlic
- 3 tablespoons extra-virgin olive oil
- 1 to 2 tablespoons tahini
- 1 to 2 tablespoons fresh lemon juice
- ¼ teaspoon salt
- 2 tablespoons water

INSTRUCTIONS

1. In a food processor, blend the chickpeas, garlic, oil, tahini, lemon juice, salt, and water until smooth.

2. Serve as a dip with whole-wheat pita bread or as a spread in sandwiches. Makes 4 servings (approximately ¼ cup per serving).

Tip! Jazz up your hummus by mixing in different flavors. For example, blend hummus with sun-dried tomatoes or mix in pine nuts or olives.

SERVING SIZE	TOTAL FAT	CHOLESTEROL	TOTAL CARBS	SUGARS
• 114 g	• 16.7	• 0 mg	• 24.8 g	• 4.3 g
CALORIES	SATURATED FAT	SODIUM	DIETARY FIBER	PROTEIN
• 272	• 2.3 g	• 356 mg	• 7 g	• 8.7 g

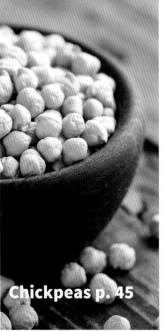

Chickpeas p. 45

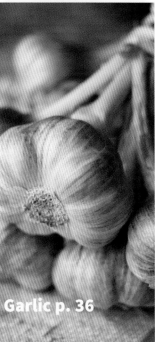

Garlic p. 36

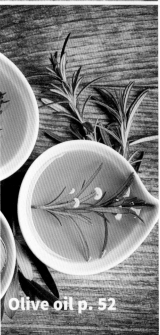

Olive oil p. 52

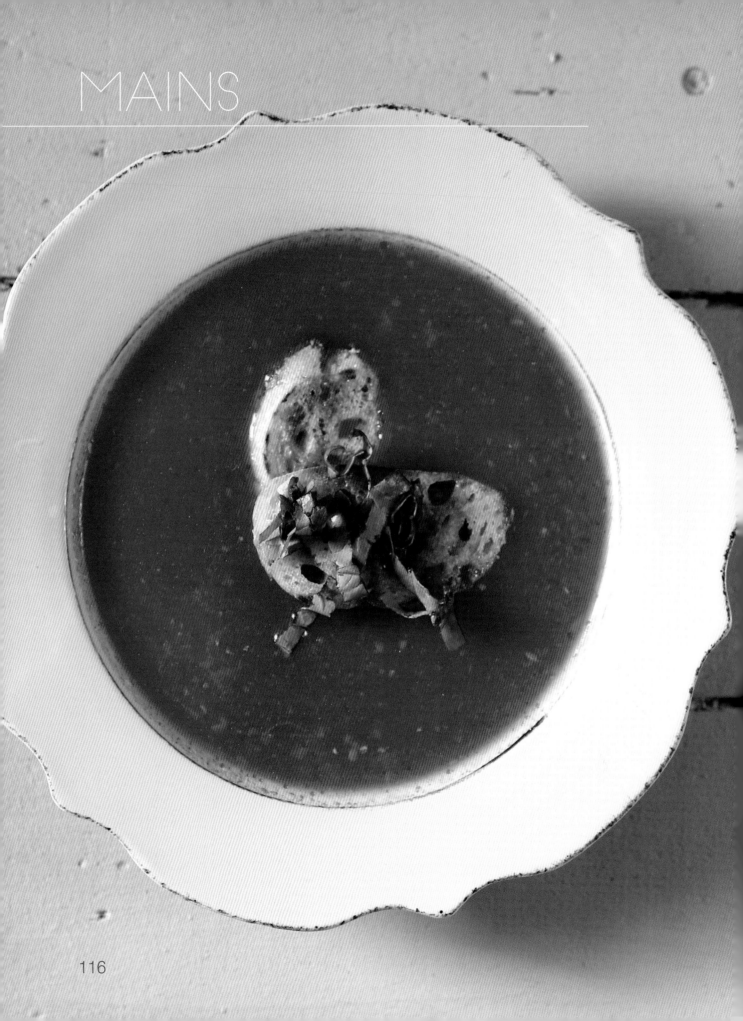

Tomato Soup

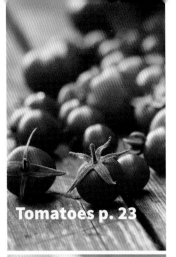

Tomatoes p. 23

INGREDIENTS

- 1 cup chopped onions
- 1 teaspoon dried basil
- 2 tablespoons olive oil
- 2 cloves garlic, minced
- 1 (13-oz) can diced tomatoes
- 1 carrot, cut into large chunks
- 3 ½ cups water, divided
- ½ teaspoon salt

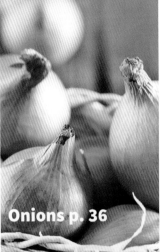

Onions p. 36

INSTRUCTIONS

1. In a medium saucepan, sauté onions and basil in olive oil for 5 to 7 minutes, then add garlic and sauté for another minute. Add diced tomatoes, carrot, and 2 cups of water. Bring mixture to a boil, reduce to a simmer, and simmer for 20 minutes.

2. Ladle mixture into a blender and blend carefully in batches. If you would like a smooth soup, blend the entire pot of soup. If you prefer a soup with some texture, blend half of the mixture. Return blended mixture to saucepan, add remaining 1 ½ cups water, bring to a boil, reduce to a simmer, and simmer an additional 20 minutes. Add salt and stir to combine. Makes 5 servings (approximately 1 cup per serving).

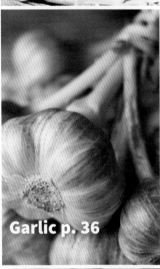

Garlic p. 36

SERVING SIZE	TOTAL FAT	CHOLESTEROL	TOTAL CARBS	SUGARS
• 288 g	• 5.6 g	• 0 mg	• 7.6 g	• 3.5 g
CALORIES	SATURATED FAT	SODIUM	DIETARY FIBER	PROTEIN
• 83	• 0.8 g	• 257 mg	• 1.5 g	• 1.1 g

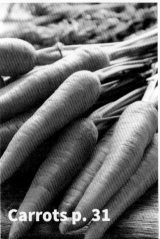

Carrots p. 31

Cancer-Fighting Ingredients

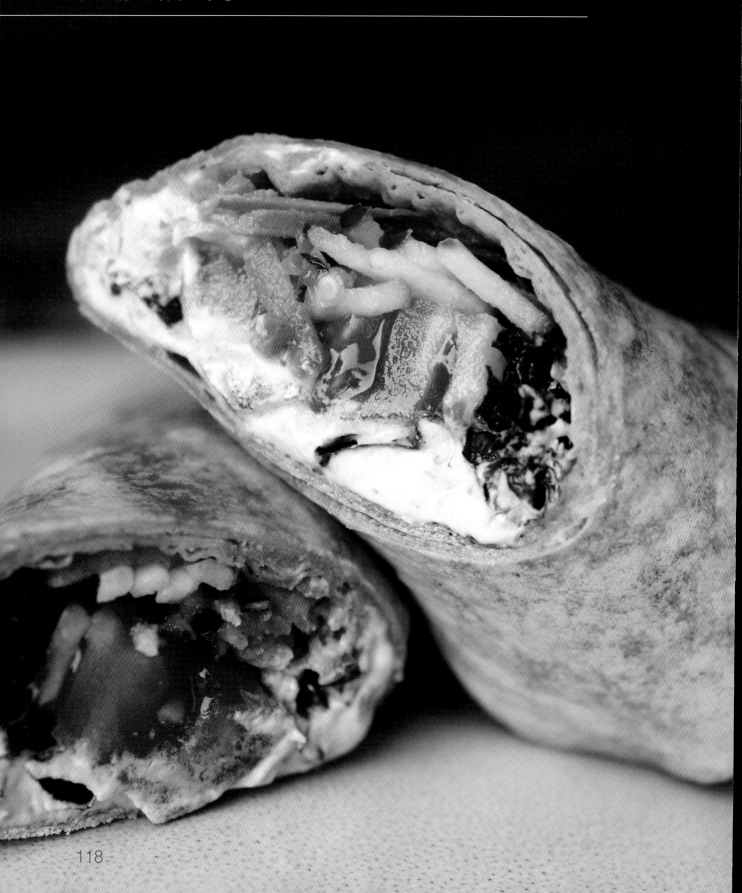

Veggie Wrap With "Cream Cheese"

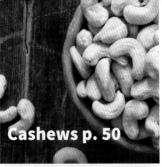
Cashews p. 50

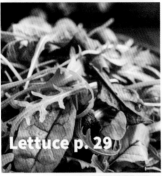
Lettuce p. 29

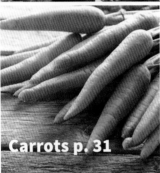
Carrots p. 31

INGREDIENTS

- 1 cup raw cashews, soaked for 2 hours or up to overnight
- ¼ cup water
- 2 tablespoons avocado oil (or other light-tasting oil)
- ¼ teaspoon salt
- 2 tablespoons fresh lemon juice
- 8 whole-wheat tortillas
- 2 cups shredded lettuce
- 1 large carrot, grated
- 1 cucumber, sliced
- 2 medium tomatoes, sliced

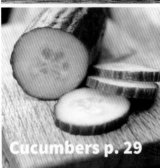
Cucumbers p. 29

INSTRUCTIONS

1. Drain and rinse the cashews and add to a blender along with water, oil, salt, and lemon juice. Blend until smooth. For best flavor, store in an airtight container in refrigerator for a few hours or overnight.

2. For each wrap, spread about 2 tablespoons of cashew "cream cheese" on tortilla, then top with lettuce, carrot, cucumber, and tomatoes. Makes 8 wraps.

Tip! Mix up the types of vegetables in your filling. Add cabbage, shredded Brussels sprouts, grated beets, whatever you like!

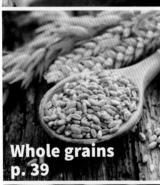
Whole grains p. 39

SERVING SIZE	TOTAL FAT	CHOLESTEROL	TOTAL CARBS	SUGARS
• 169 g	• 11.2 g	• 0 mg	• 30.4 g	• 3.1 g
CALORIES	SATURATED FAT	SODIUM	DIETARY FIBER	PROTEIN
• 243	• 1.6 g	• 214 mg	• 4.4 g	• 7.2 g

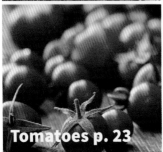
Tomatoes p. 23

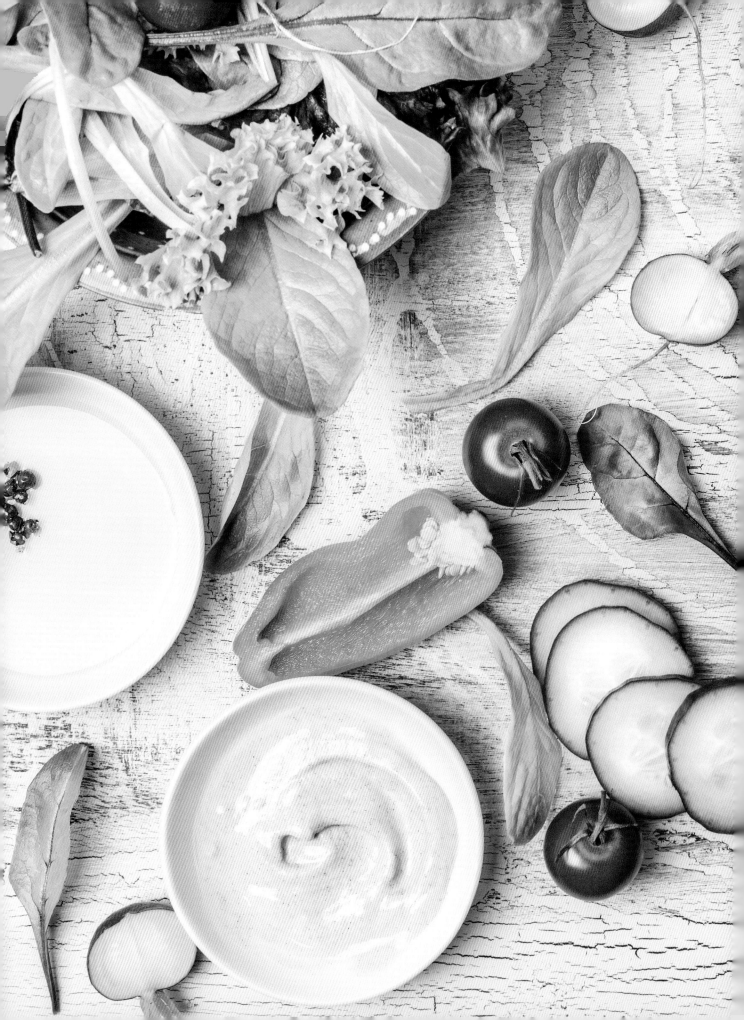

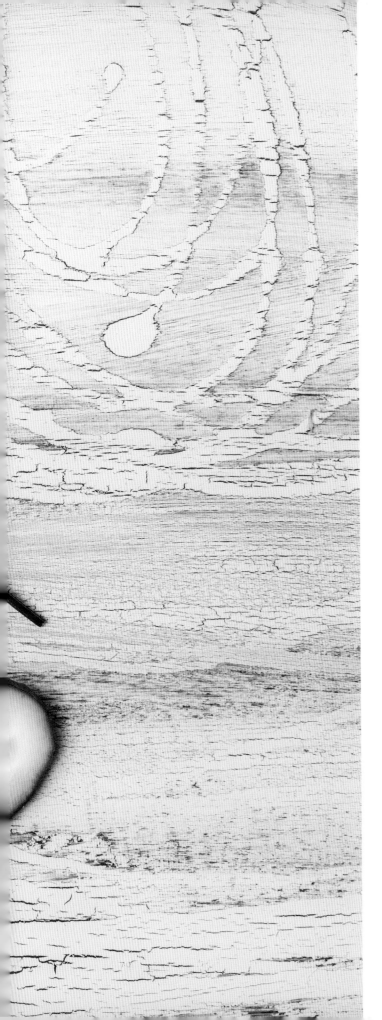

Salads

Cilantro Citrus Slaw

Romaine Salad With Creamy Walnut Dressing

Broccoli Salad

SALADS

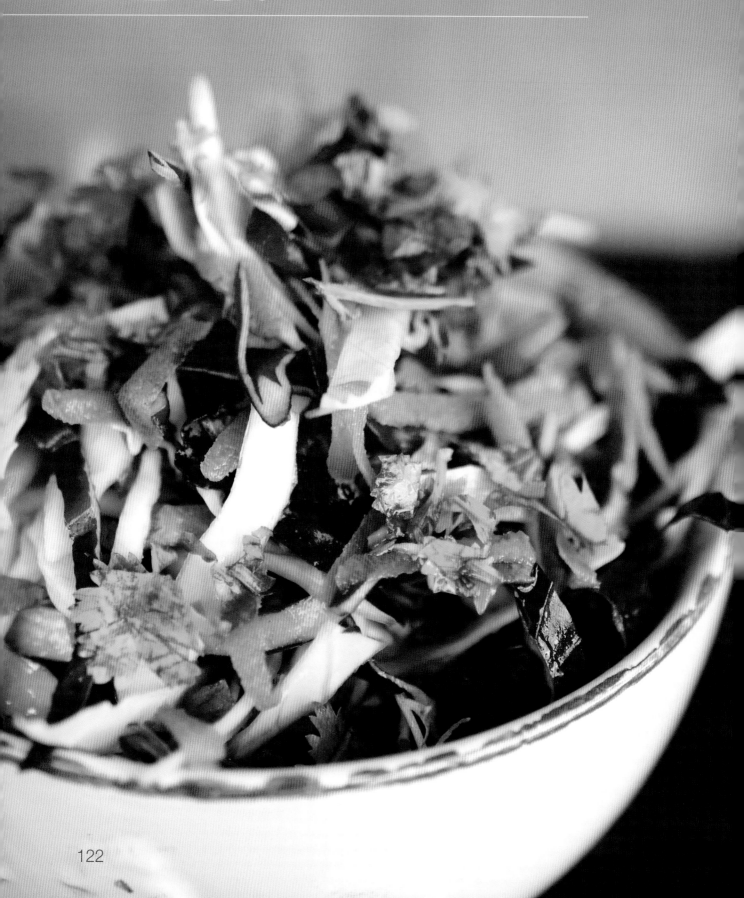

Cilantro Citrus Slaw

INGREDIENTS

- ¼ cup fresh orange juice
- 3 tablespoons extra-virgin olive oil
- ¼ teaspoon salt
- 1 teaspoon honey
- 1 clove garlic, finely minced
- 1 cup shredded red cabbage
- 1 cup shredded green cabbage
- 1 cup grated carrots
- ½ cup finely chopped fresh cilantro

INSTRUCTIONS

1. In a bowl, whisk together orange juice, olive oil, salt, honey, and garlic. In a larger bowl, combine red cabbage, green cabbage, carrots, and cilantro.

2. Add dressing to slaw mixture and toss to combine. Makes 6 servings (approximately ½ cup per serving).

SERVING SIZE	TOTAL FAT	CHOLESTEROL	TOTAL CARBS	SUGARS
• 63 g	• 7.1 g	• 0 mg	• 5.6 g	• 3.6 g
CALORIES	SATURATED FAT	SODIUM	DIETARY FIBER	PROTEIN
• 83	• 1 g	• 116 mg	• 1.1 g	• 0.6 g

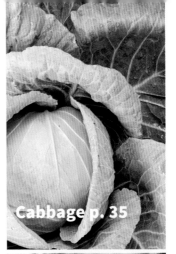

Cabbage p. 35

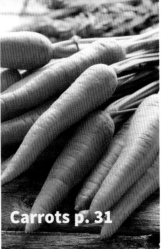

Carrots p. 31

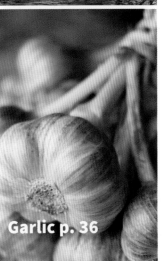

Garlic p. 36

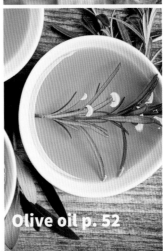

Olive oil p. 52

Cancer-Fighting Ingredients

SALADS

Romaine Salad With Creamy Walnut Dressing

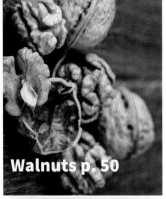

Walnuts p. 50

INGREDIENTS

- ¾ cup raw walnuts
- ¼ cup raw cashews
- 2 tablespoons extra-virgin olive oil
- 1 to 2 cloves garlic
- 12 pitted olives
- ¼ cup plus 2 tablespoons water
- ¼ teaspoon salt*
- Romaine lettuce
- Chopped walnuts for topping

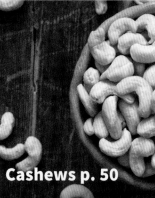

Cashews p. 50

INSTRUCTIONS

1. In a blender, blend walnuts, cashews, oil, garlic, olives, water, and salt until smooth. Add 2 tablespoons of dressing for every 2 cups of romaine lettuce, and toss to combine.

2. Top salad with chopped walnuts if desired. Makes 10 servings of salad (2 cups romaine lettuce plus 2 tablespoons dressing).

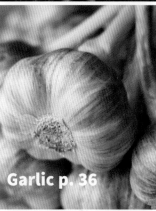

Garlic p. 36

NOTE:

* If your olives are salty, omit ¼ teaspoon salt.

SERVING SIZE	TOTAL FAT	CHOLESTEROL	TOTAL CARBS	SUGARS
121 g	10.8 g	0 mg	5.2 g	1.1 g
CALORIES	SATURATED FAT	SODIUM	DIETARY FIBER	PROTEIN
125	1.1 g	96 mg	3.1 g	3.3 g

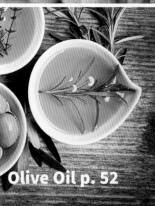

Olive Oil p. 52

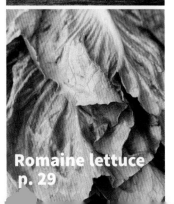

Romaine lettuce p. 29

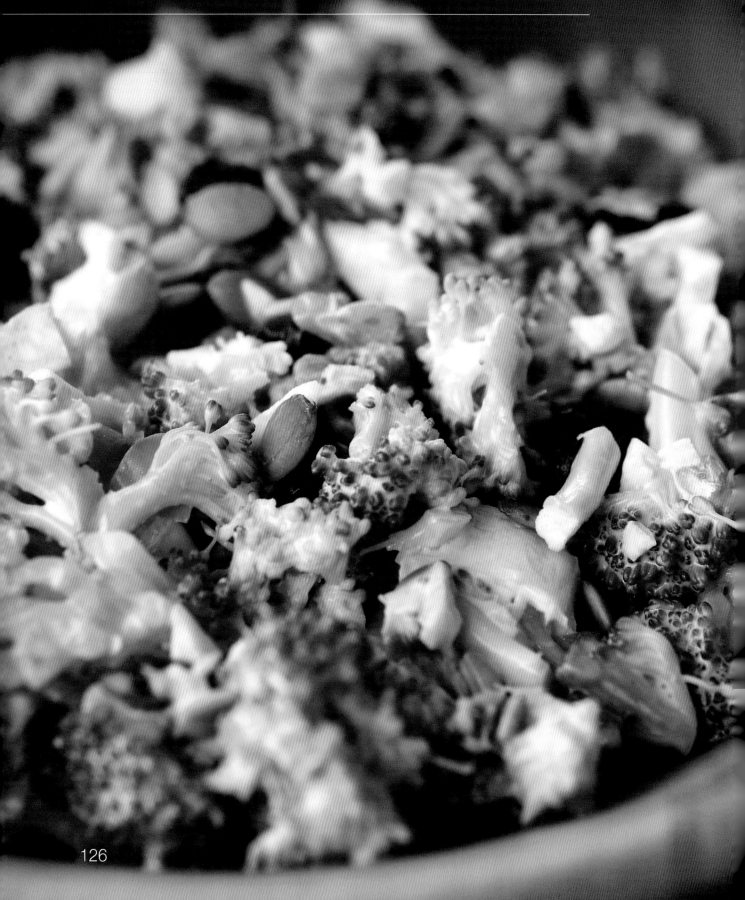

Broccoli Salad

INGREDIENTS

- ¼ cup avocado oil (or other light-tasting oil)
- ¼ cup cold unsweetened soy milk
- 1 teaspoon honey
- ¼ teaspoon salt
- 4 cups finely chopped broccoli
- ½ cup mixed nuts, seeds, and dried fruit

INSTRUCTIONS

1. In a blender, blend oil, soy milk, honey, and salt until well blended. Mixture should resemble mayonnaise but if it doesn't, that's OK.

2. Add broccoli and mixed nuts, seeds, and dried fruit to a large bowl, then add dressing. Mix well. Makes 8 servings (approximately ½ cup per serving).

SERVING SIZE	TOTAL FAT	CHOLESTEROL	TOTAL CARBS	SUGARS
• 68 g	• 8.8 g	• 0 mg	• 7.3 g	• 3.8 g
CALORIES	SATURATED FAT	SODIUM	DIETARY FIBER	PROTEIN
• 113	• 1.1 g	• 101 mg	• 1.7 g	• 2.2 g

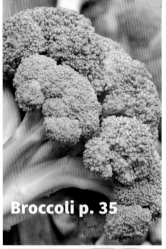

Broccoli p. 35

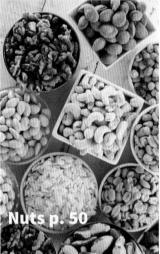

Nuts p. 50

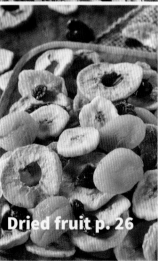

Dried fruit p. 26

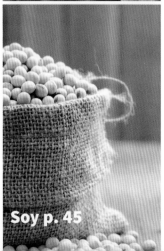

Soy p. 45

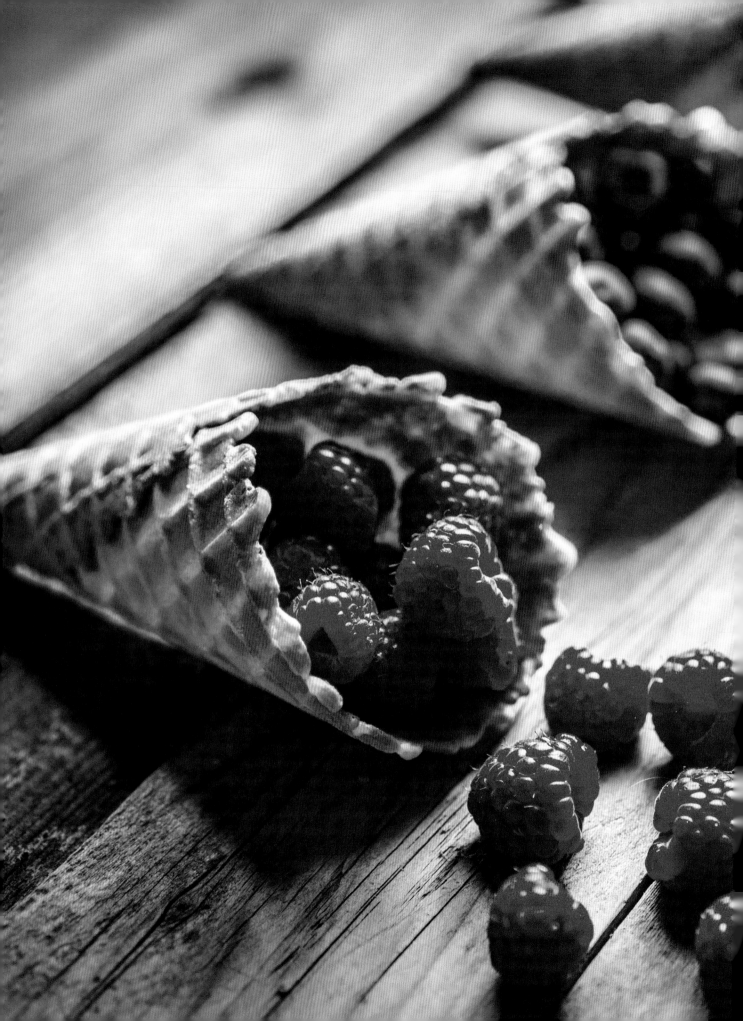

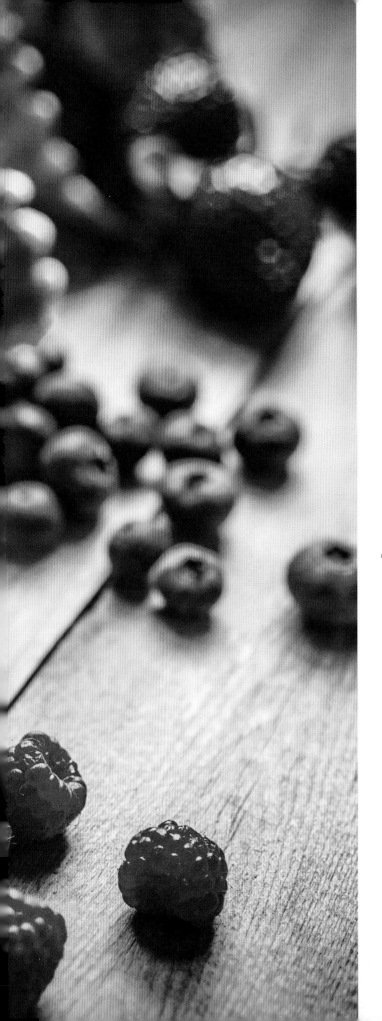

Sweet Treats

Baked Peaches

Oatmeal-Walnut Cookies

Banana Ice Cream

Crispy Sunflower Bars

Grape-Pomegranate Sorbet

Carrot Cake

Fruit Parfait

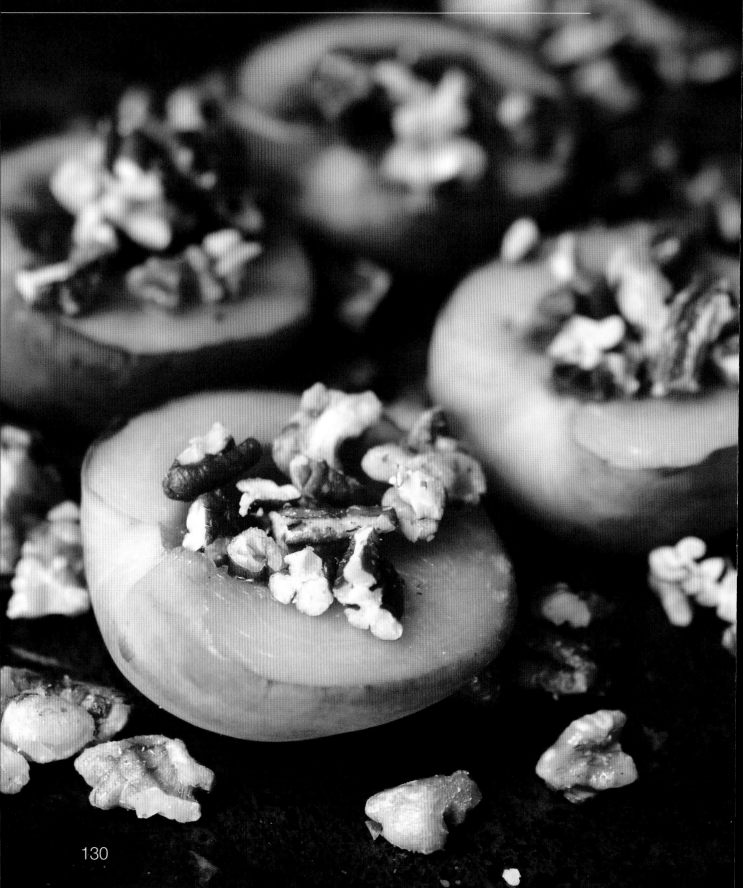

Baked Peaches

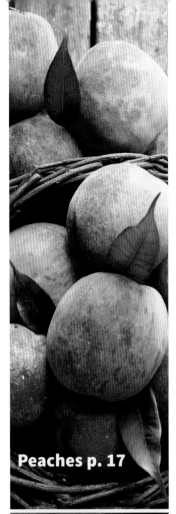

INGREDIENTS

- 4 peaches
- 4 teaspoons honey
- 1 cup toasted walnuts

INSTRUCTIONS

1. Preheat oven to 350 degrees Fahrenheit. Wash peaches and cut them in half, removing the pits. Lightly brush each peach with 1 teaspoon honey and bake for 10 to 15 minutes, or until peaches are softened and warmed through.

2. Top peaches with toasted walnuts. You may add a little nondairy whipped topping or some vegan ice cream if desired. Makes 4 servings.

SERVING SIZE	TOTAL FAT	CHOLESTEROL	TOTAL CARBS	SUGARS
180 g	15.2 g	0 mg	18.2 g	13.3 g

CALORIES	SATURATED FAT	SODIUM	DIETARY FIBER	PROTEIN
208	1.5 g	0.2 mg	3.4 g	4.5 g

Peaches p. 17

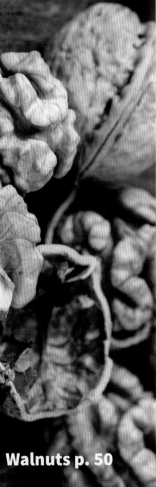

Walnuts p. 50

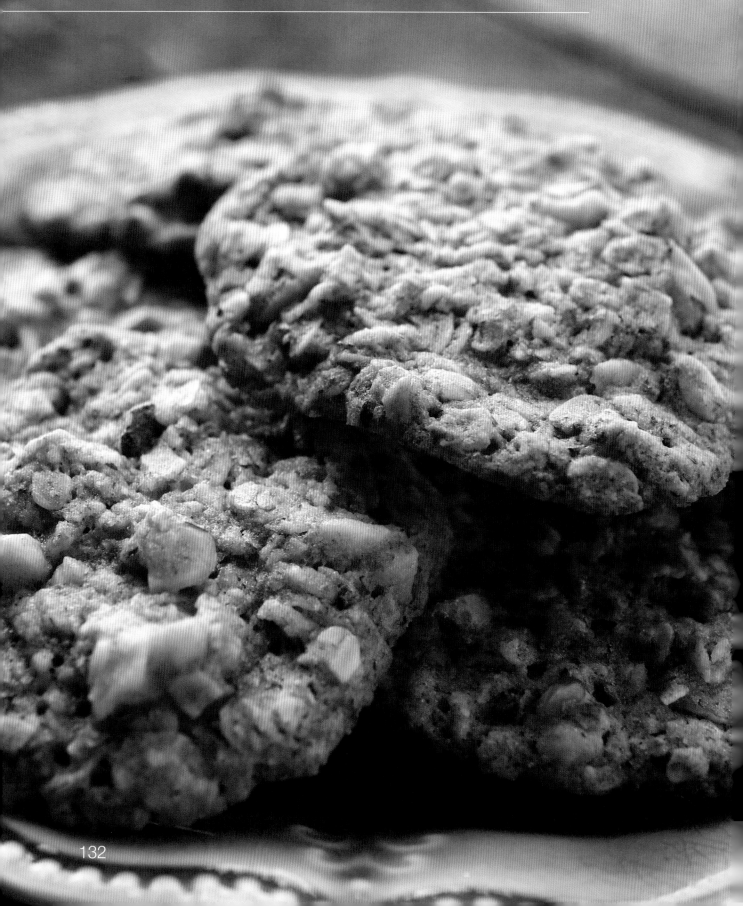

Oatmeal-Walnut Cookies

INGREDIENTS

- 1 cup whole-wheat flour
- 2 tablespoons ground flaxseeds
- ¼ teaspoon salt
- ½ teaspoon baking soda
- ¾ cup solid unrefined coconut oil
- ¾ cup honey
- 2 cups rolled oats
- 1 cup chopped raw walnuts

INSTRUCTIONS

1. In a large bowl, combine flour, ground flaxseeds, salt, and baking soda and stir. Add coconut oil and mix into the flour mixture until completely mixed in and there are no chunks or pieces of coconut oil (you may use a food processor to cut coconut oil into flour mixture as well). Mixture will resemble wet sand. Add honey to flour and coconut oil mixture and mix well, then add rolled oats and mix until evenly combined. Finally, add chopped walnuts and mix until combined.

2. Preheat oven to 350 degrees Fahrenheit. Line 2 baking trays with parchment paper (you may need to bake cookies in a couple of batches). Divide cookie dough into 2-tablespoon portions, form each portion into a ball, slightly flatten it, and set it on the lined baking tray, keeping the cookies at least 1 ½ inches apart. Bake cookies for 12 to 15 minutes, or until tops are light golden brown. Remove baking tray from oven and gently transfer parchment paper with the cookies to the counter, or gently transfer cookies to a cooling rack (cookies will be very soft fresh out of the oven). Allow cookies to cool for at least 10 minutes. Makes 28 cookies.

Tip! To help prevent the bottom of the cookies from over-browning, bake them on aluminum baking sheets as darker baking sheets tend to cause cookies to brown faster. Alternatively, line darker baking sheets with aluminum foil, then place parchment paper on top of foil. Also try placing an empty baking tray or a sheet of aluminum foil on the rack just below your rack of cookies so cookies have some protection from direct heat.

SERVING SIZE	TOTAL FAT	CHOLESTEROL	TOTAL CARBS	SUGARS
30 g	9.6 g	0 mg	15.8 g	7.6 g
CALORIES	SATURATED FAT	SODIUM	DIETARY FIBER	PROTEIN
159	5.9 g	42 mg	1.6 g	2.4 g

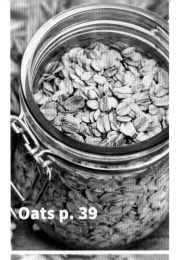

Oats p. 39

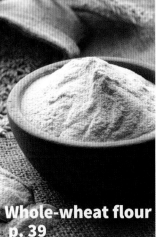

Whole-wheat flour p. 39

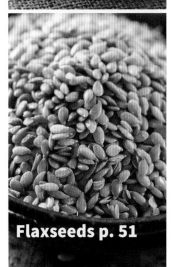

Flaxseeds p. 51

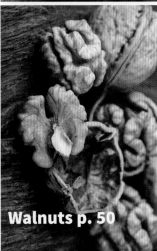

Walnuts p. 50

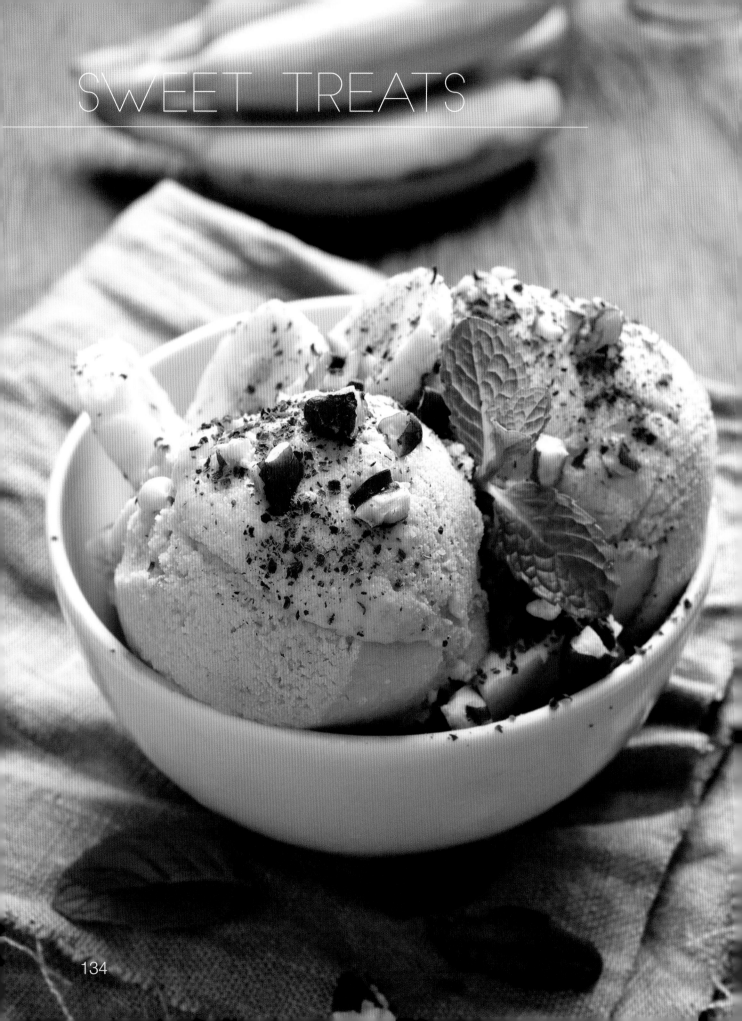

Banana Ice Cream

INGREDIENTS

- 6 bananas
- Berries (optional)

INSTRUCTIONS

1. Peel, dice, and freeze bananas for at least 2 hours or overnight. Process them in a food processor for instant, smooth ice cream.

2. For different flavors, add other fruits like frozen strawberries or blueberries. Makes 4 servings.

SERVING SIZE	TOTAL FAT	CHOLESTEROL	TOTAL CARBS	SUGARS
• 177 g	• 0.6 g	• 0 mg	• 40.4 g	• 21.7 g
CALORIES	SATURATED FAT	SODIUM	DIETARY FIBER	PROTEIN
• 158	• 0.2 g	• 2 mg	• 4.6 g	• 1.9 g

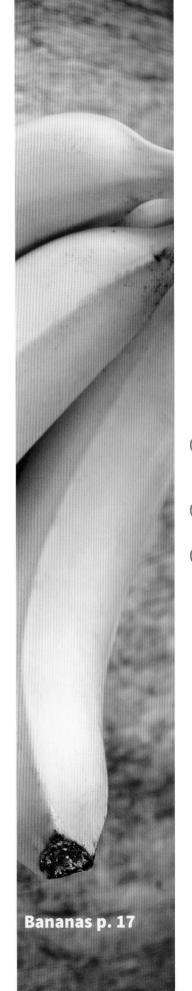

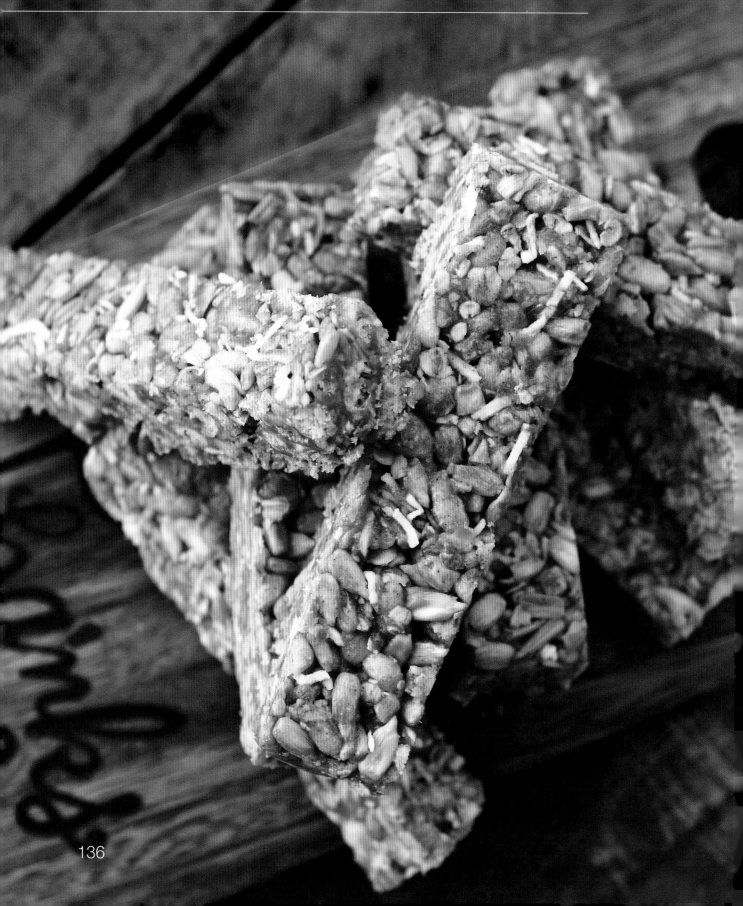

Crispy Sunflower Bars

INGREDIENTS

- 1 ¾ cups brown crispy rice cereal*
- 1 cup raw sunflower seeds
- ½ cup quick oats
- ½ cup shredded unsweetened coconut
- ¾ cup smooth unsalted and unsweetened peanut butter**
- ¼ cup honey
- ¼ teaspoon salt
- 1 teaspoon vanilla extract

INSTRUCTIONS

1. In a large bowl, combine rice cereal, sunflower seeds, quick oats, and coconut and stir. In a smaller bowl, combine peanut butter, honey, and salt and mix well. Pour peanut butter mixture into cereal mixture and mix well.

2. Spread mixture evenly into a 9x9-inches square baking pan and press firmly. Freeze for 1 to 2 hours. Loosen sides of cereal mixture by running a metal spatula around the sides, then carefully overturn mixture onto a cutting board. Alternatively, cut directly in pan. Using a sharp serrated knife, cut cereal mixture into 16 rectangular bars. Store bars in freezer. Makes 16 pieces.

NOTE:

* May be substituted with other puffed rice cereal (such as Kellogg's Rice Krispies) if brown crispy rice cereal is difficult to find

** May be substituted with another nut or seed butter of your choice

SERVING SIZE	TOTAL FAT	CHOLESTEROL	TOTAL CARBS	SUGARS
33 g	12.4 g	0 mg	12.4 g	5.4 g
CALORIES	SATURATED FAT	SODIUM	DIETARY FIBER	PROTEIN
180	3.3 g	41 mg	2.3 g	5.4 g

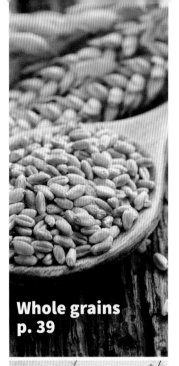

Whole grains p. 39

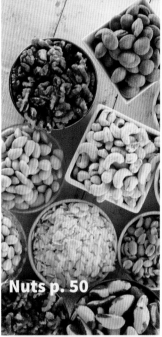

Nuts p. 50

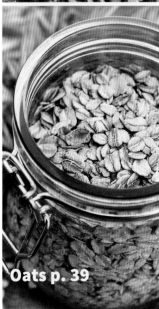

Oats p. 39

Cancer-Fighting Ingredients

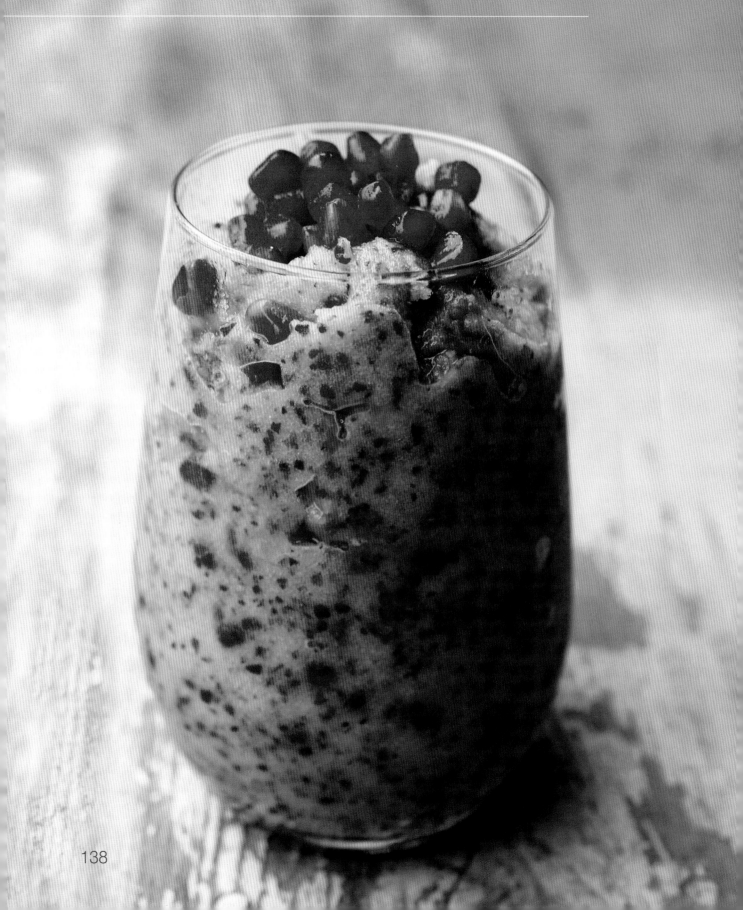

Grape-Pomegranate Sorbet

INGREDIENTS

- 5 cups grapes
- 1 cup pomegranate seeds

INSTRUCTIONS

1. Wash grapes well, then freeze for at least 4 hours or overnight. When grapes are completely frozen, process them in a food processor until smooth.

2. Mix in pomegranate seeds, and reserve a few seeds to garnish. Serve immediately. Makes 4 servings.

SERVING SIZE	TOTAL FAT	CHOLESTEROL	TOTAL CARBS	SUGARS
• 159 g	• 0.7 g	• 0 mg	• 23.7 g	• 21.7 g
CALORIES	SATURATED FAT	SODIUM	DIETARY FIBER	PROTEIN
• 95	• 0.1 g	• 3 mg	• 1.8 g	• 1 g

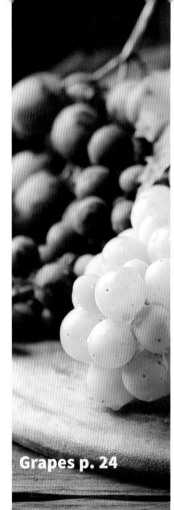

Grapes p. 24

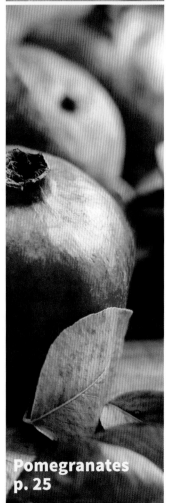

Pomegranates p. 25

Cancer-Fighting Ingredients

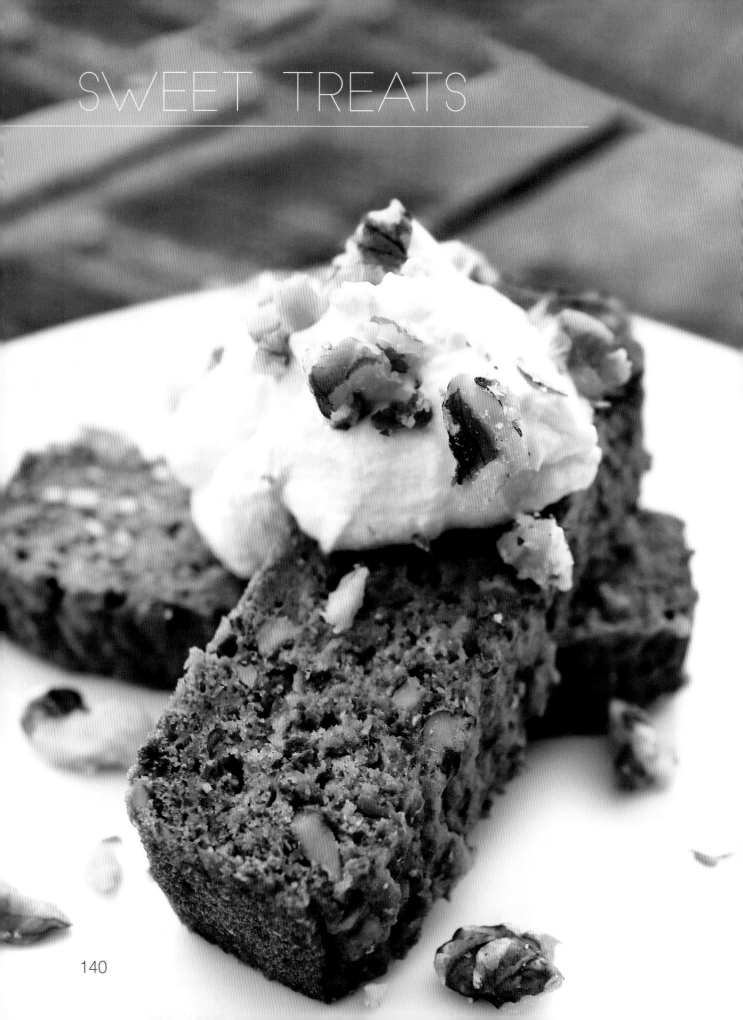

SWEET TREATS

Carrot Cake

INGREDIENTS

- 2 cups whole-wheat flour
- 1 cup finely chopped walnuts
- ¼ cup ground flaxseeds
- 2 teaspoons baking powder
- ½ teaspoon baking soda
- ¼ teaspoon salt
- 2 cups finely grated carrots
- 2 apples
- ½ cup honey
- 12 pitted dates
- 1 cup unsweetened soy milk
- ⅓ cup avocado oil (or other light-tasting oil)
- 1 teaspoon vanilla extract

INSTRUCTIONS

1. In a large bowl combine flour, walnuts, flaxseeds, baking powder, baking soda, and salt. Mix until well combined, then add grated carrots and mix until carrots are evenly distributed through flour. Remove core from apples, chop apples in large chunks (do not peel), and add to a blender along with honey, dates, soy milk, oil, and vanilla. Blend until smooth.

2. Add blended mixture to flour mixture and stir just until the batter is evenly mixed and there is no more dry flour. Do not overmix. Pour batter into a 9-inch round or 8x8-inch or 9x9-inch square cake pan and bake at 350 degrees Fahrenheit for 35 to 45 minutes, or until a toothpick inserted into the center comes out clean. Makes 16 pieces.

SERVING SIZE	TOTAL FAT	CHOLESTEROL	TOTAL CARBS	SUGARS
99 g	10.7 g	0 mg	31.1 g	16.1 g
CALORIES	SATURATED FAT	SODIUM	DIETARY FIBER	PROTEIN
227	1.3 g	87 mg	3.5 g	4.4 g

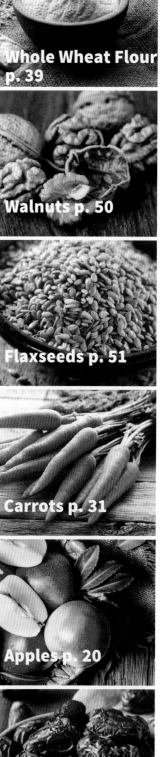

Whole Wheat Flour p. 39

Walnuts p. 50

Flaxseeds p. 51

Carrots p. 31

Apples p. 20

Dates p. 26

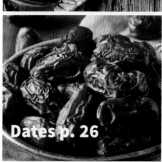

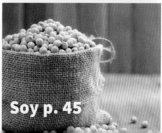

Soy p. 45

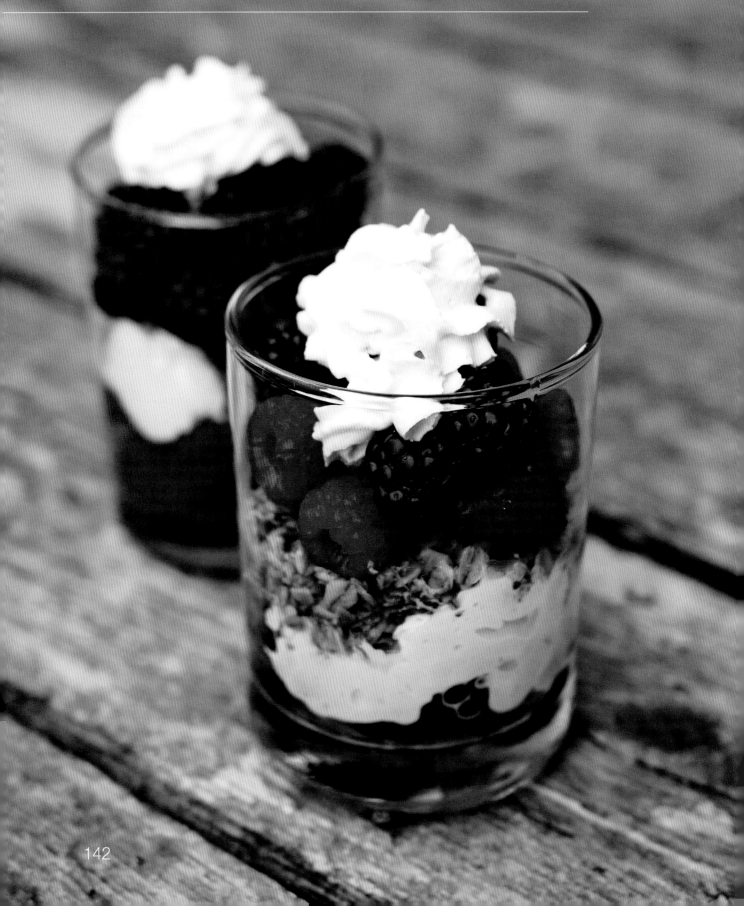

Fruit Parfait

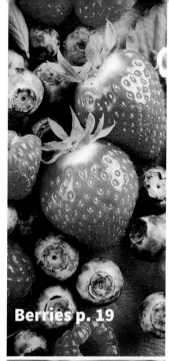

Berries p. 19

INGREDIENTS

- 4 cups fresh mixed berries
- 1 cup granola
- 1 cup nondairy whipped topping

INSTRUCTIONS

1. Set out 4 glasses. To the bottom of each glass add ½ cup mixed berries. Then add 2 tablespoons nondairy whipped topping of your choice. Then add 2 tablespoons granola.

2. Add another ½ cup berries on top, then another 2 tablespoons nondairy whipped topping, and top with another 2 tablespoons granola. Repeat for the other glasses and serve immediately. Makes 4 servings.

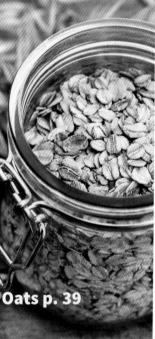

Oats p. 39

SERVING SIZE	TOTAL FAT	CHOLESTEROL	TOTAL CARBS	SUGARS
234 g	9.9 g	0 mg	39.2 g	12 g
CALORIES	SATURATED FAT	SODIUM	DIETARY FIBER	PROTEIN
262	3.3 g	8.5 mg	7.8 g	7.5 g

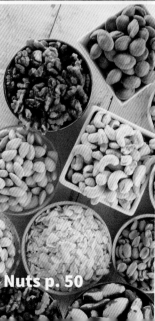

Nuts p. 50

Cancer-Fighting Ingredients

Beyond the Plate

Take care of your body. It's the only
place you have to live.
—Jim Rohn

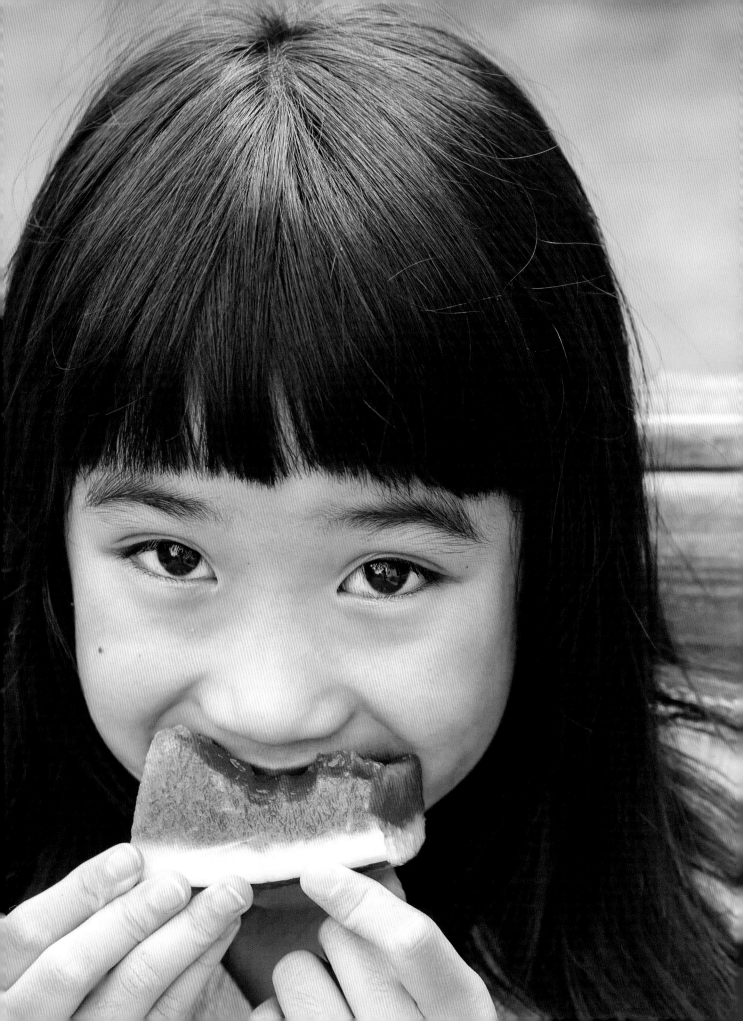

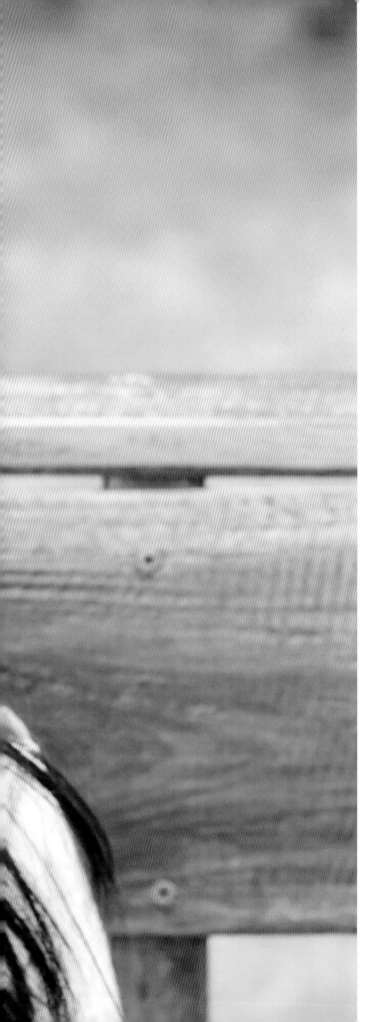

It Begins With Eight

Laws play a critical role in ordered, healthy societies. They identify things we should or should not do to maintain the safety and happiness of all. Laws govern how we drive, how we educate, and how we keep the peace. They determine food safety, water quality, environmental health, and societal integrity. Without laws, society would be at risk and would disintegrate into mass confusion.

Our bodies are like small societies. The cells that make up our various organs grow, reproduce, and carry out various tasks. They act as busy workers, performing functions that keep us alive. So how do we keep them healthy? Fortunately, the answer is simple, and it begins with eight.

There are eight laws that form the building blocks of a healthy body. These laws are simple, practical, and available to all. Even better, if you put them into practice, they will help ensure that your body runs as smoothly as possible, for as long as possible.

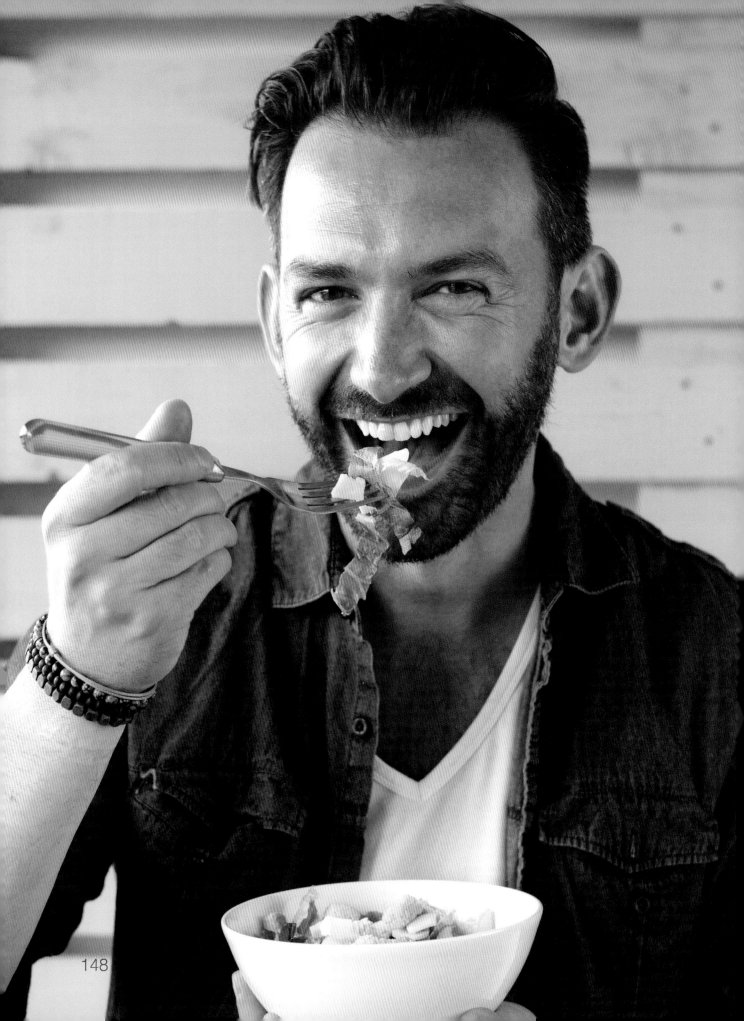

Nutrition

Our cells are the building blocks of our bodies. They are also the foundational centers of the many biological processes we depend on from day to day. They need fuel to do their work, and that fuel comes from the food we eat. Nutrition is all about eating foods that promote health and avoiding foods that are harmful. The quality of the food is important because it dictates the health of our cells and ultimately, of our bodies. Just as a car needs the right kind of fuel to perform at its best, we need the right kind of fuel to perform at our best.

Timing Is Everything

It is said that we should eat breakfast like a king, lunch like a queen, and dinner like a pauper. As it happens, research finds strong support for this idea. Our bodies are ordered and regulated through the activities of "clocks" scattered throughout our various cells. Our adrenal glands have clocks. Our lungs have clocks. Our spleens have clocks. Even our pancreas has a clock. And all these clocks set ideal times for ideal functions. When we respect these times, we help our bodies function normally. When we disregard them, whether by irregular eating or sleeping, we promote dysfunction and disease.

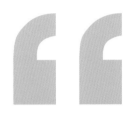

Our bodies work best when we follow the king-queen-pauper recommendation. One of the many benefits we experience is weight loss. One study found that individuals who eat most of their calories in the morning and afternoon lose *significantly more weight* than those who eat most of their calories in the evening,[174] *even when the same amount of calories are consumed*.[175] Why is this important for cancer? Because approximately 20 percent of all cancer cases are attributable to weight gain and obesity.[176] One study has said that "overeating may be the largest avoidable cause of cancer in non-smokers."[177] If we eat at appropriate times, our bodies can better help us lose excess weight. This in turn helps reduce our cancer risk.

Consistently eating at regular times is also important. One study found that those who ate their meals at regular times experienced

- improved metabolism;
- lower cholesterol levels; and
- improved insulin response.[178]

On the other hand, eating at irregular times causes a number of problems. These include insulin resistance, which increases the risk of cardiovascular disease.[179]

So what is the takeaway? When it comes to nutrition, *when* you eat is just as important as *what* you eat. Eat most of your calories in the morning and afternoon, and reduce or eliminate evening calorie consumption. Additionally, be consistent with your mealtimes. Once you have come up with a meal schedule that fits your needs, do everything possible to stick to it.

> When it comes to nutrition, *when* you eat is just as important as *what* you eat.

Snack Attack

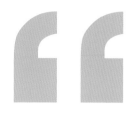

Eating frequent meals throughout the day is often promoted as a strategy for managing weight loss. But one study done in 2015 made a remarkable observation:

"At present, there is still a perception within the general community, and amongst some nutritionists, that eating multiple small meals spaced throughout the day is beneficial for weight control and metabolic health. However, *intervention trials do not generally support the epidemiological evidence*, and data is emerging to suggest that *increasing the fasting period between meals may beneficially impact body weight and metabolic health*."[180]

A number of studies have found that snacking actually *hinders* weight loss because it hijacks mechanisms within our bodies that control the storage and burning of fat. For example, studies have shown that:

- Snacking promotes the storage of fat cells. This is because when you constantly eat, your body keeps your insulin levels elevated, and insulin causes fat to be stored.[181]

- Patients who eat two meals a day, early in the day, have better health outcomes than those who eat six meals, *even though both groups eat the same amount of calories*. In the study, one group of patients with type 2 diabetes was given two meals a day, breakfast and lunch. The other group received six meals. The group that ate two meals reduced their weight, liver fat content, and fasting glucose levels more than those who ate six meals. This was true even though both groups ate the same amount of calories.[182]

As mentioned earlier, snacking keeps the level of insulin in your blood constantly elevated. This causes other problems, including hypertension and cardiovascular issues. This is because elevated insulin promotes the production of LDL (bad) cholesterol.[183] Insulin is also atherogenic. This means it promotes the transportation and deposit of cholesterol onto the walls of our arteries.[184] So the more insulin is in our bloodstream, the more cholesterol is being deposited into our arteries, and this leads to cardiovascular problems.

While constant snacking causes a number of problems, allowing extended periods of rest between meals does good things for the body. It helps improve mental function,[185] cardiovascular health, diabetes management, longevity, and overall health.[186] This is because these rest periods reduce damage to our cells from free radicals and increase our cells' ability to fight stress.[187]

Eating the right things at the right time maximizes our bodies' natural functions and minimizes strain. This brings a world of benefits, including weight loss. So when it comes to snacking, the best advice is to refrain. The saying goes, "Eat breakfast like a king, lunch like a queen, and supper like a pauper." There is no mention of snacks, and that may very well be the point.

When it comes to snacking, the best advice is to refrain. The saying goes, "Eat breakfast like a king, lunch like a queen, and supper like a pauper." There is no mention of snacks, and that may very well be the point.

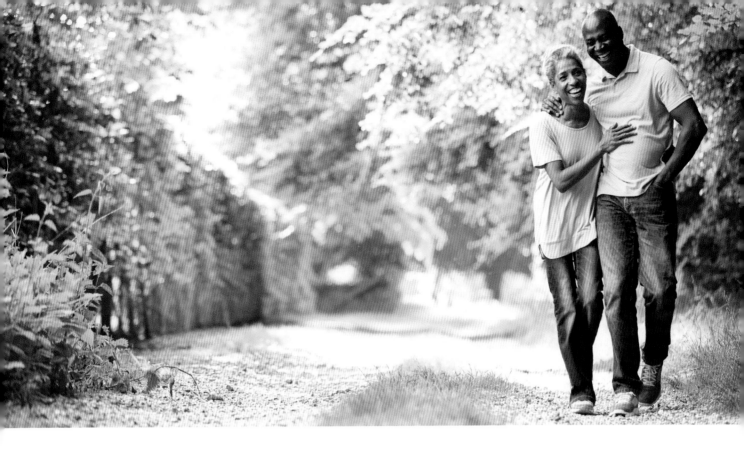

Walk It Off

It may seem strange to find information about walking in a section about nutrition, but research has found that walking is not just about exercise. It also has a part to play in good digestion. Studies show that taking a short, easy walk after a meal

- regulates blood sugar after eating carbohydrates and prevents a blood sugar spike;[188]

- helps the stomach empty its contents more quickly,[189] improving digestion; and

- helps prevent heartburn that is connected with delayed emptying of stomach contents.[190]

So if you want to make the most of your food, take 15 minutes after each meal to walk off sugar spikes and heartburn and other forms of indigestion.

RECOMMENDATIONS:

- Eat a diet rich in fruits, vegetables, and whole grains.
- Get plenty of fiber in your diet. Good sources are beans, whole grains, fruits, and vegetables.
- Eat healthy fats, such as those founds in nuts, seeds, olives, and avocados.
- Avoid overeating.
- Minimize or avoid the use of animal products, such as meats and dairy.
- Use salt and added sugar sparingly.
- Minimize or avoid spicy foods and condiments.
- Eat at regular times, and allow your stomach to rest for at least five hours between mealtimes.
- Follow the king-queen-pauper meal plan. For maximum health, skip the evening meal altogether. If you must eat it, eat early and eat light.
- Take a fifteen-minute walk after each meal to control blood sugar and improve digestion.

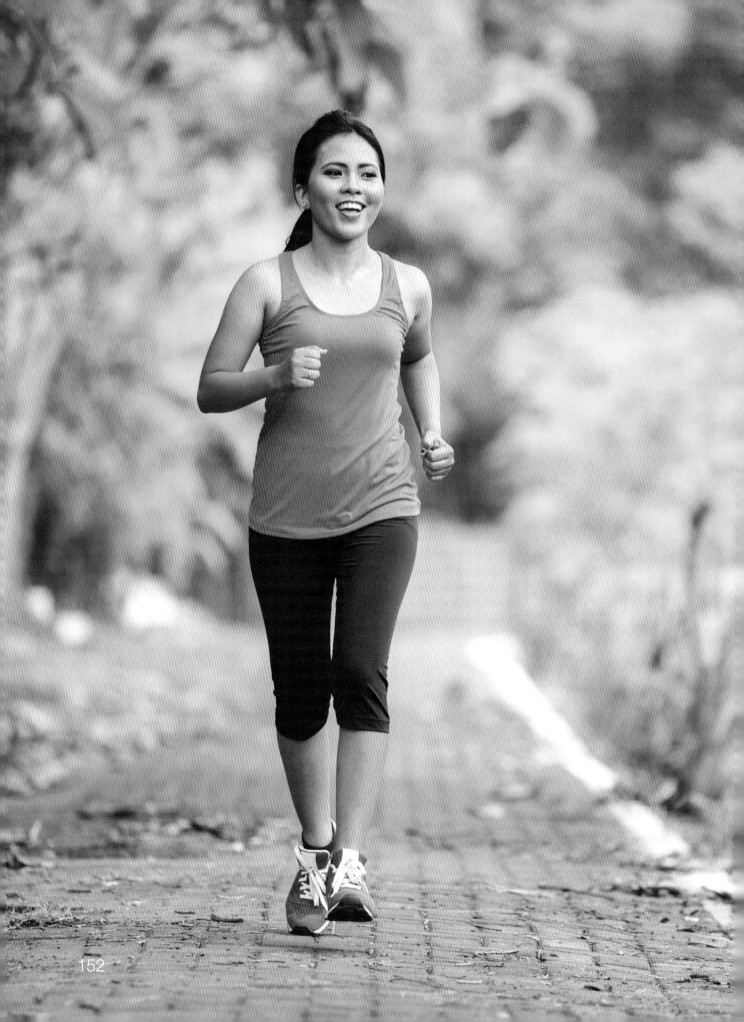

Exercise

Our bodies were designed to move. From bones to muscles to the brain that controls it all, our bodies were built to be active. So when we exercise, our bodies stay healthy and happy.

Our bones and muscles, including our heart muscle, need exercise to gain strength. When we exercise, our hearts grow stronger and pump blood more efficiently. This keeps our cells clean and well fed because the blood delivers oxygen and nutrients and removes waste. Exercise also helps ensure our cells live longer by reducing cellular stress, which shortens the life of a cell.[191]

When we exercise, our brains release chemicals that improve our mood and combat stress. Exercise also helps our brains grow and develop new neurological connections. This in turn improves memory and brain function.[192]

Exercise in Cancer Prevention and Treatment

Exercise plays an important role in cancer prevention and treatment as demonstrated in the following studies:

- Individuals who are more physically active reduce their risk of colon cancer by 24 percent compared with those who are less physically active.[193]
- Women who engage in physical activity reduce their risk of breast cancer by 25–30 percent,[194] and African American women who engage in two or more hours a week of vigorous physical activity experience a 64 percent reduced risk of breast cancer compared with those who do not engage in any physical activity.[195]
- Men who exercise reduce their risk of prostate cancer by 10–30 percent.[196]
- Women who have breast cancer and engage in regular physical activity reduce their risk of death or breast cancer recurrence.[197]
- Men who have prostate cancer and are physically active reduce their risk of dying from the cancer.[198]

RECOMMENDATIONS:

- Try 15–20 minutes of physical activity every day, and build up from there. Even as little as 15 minutes of physical activity a day provides health benefits and is a great place to start.
- Work up to 30 minutes of moderate exercise a day, five or more days a week.
- For optimal health and cancer-fighting benefits, engage in 30–60 minutes of moderate to vigorous physical activity every day.

> Our bodies were designed to move. From bones to muscles to the brain that controls it all, our bodies were built to be active. So when we exercise, our bodies stay healthy and happy.

As much as 60 percent of the adult human body is composed of water, and water makes up 73 percent of our brain and heart and 83 percent of our lungs.[199] The sheer volume of water in the human body gives some indication of just how important it is to health. Humans can survive for weeks without food, but without water, we would die in a matter of days. We need water to dissolve waste and remove it from the body and to help our cells engage in important chemical reactions.[200] We need water for digestion, temperature regulation, and lubrication.[201] Because of the vital role water plays in the health of our bodies, inadequate water intake causes a number of problems. These include headaches, poor heart function, blood pressure complications, poor kidney function, constipation, delirium, depression, reduction in cognitive performance, and fatigue.[202]

A number of studies have linked water intake to reduced cancer risk:

- Men who drink six or more cups of water a day reduce their risk of bladder cancer by 51 percent compared with those who drink less than one cup each day.[203]
- Water intake alone reduces the risk of colon cancer among women.[204]

Hydrotherapy, which uses water to treat certain medical conditions, has been used to bring relief to people suffering from pain and conditions like burns and arthritis.[205] A number of studies have also looked into its potential benefits in cancer treatment.

Hyperthermia is the carefully controlled use of heat, whether through heated water in hydrotherapy or other heat sources. It has been found to weaken cancer cells and make them more vulnerable to radiation and chemotherapy.[206] Additionally, tolerable levels of hyperthermia applied to specific regions of the body have helped delay tumor growth and promote tumor regression.[207]

> Men who drink six or more cups of water a day reduce their risk of bladder cancer by 51 percent compared with those who drink less than one cup each day.

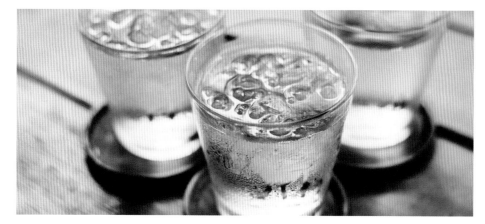

RECOMMENDATIONS:

- Drink at least 8–10 glasses of pure water every day (8 ounces per glass).
- Speak with your healthcare provider about the benefits and risks of hyperthermia in cancer treatment.

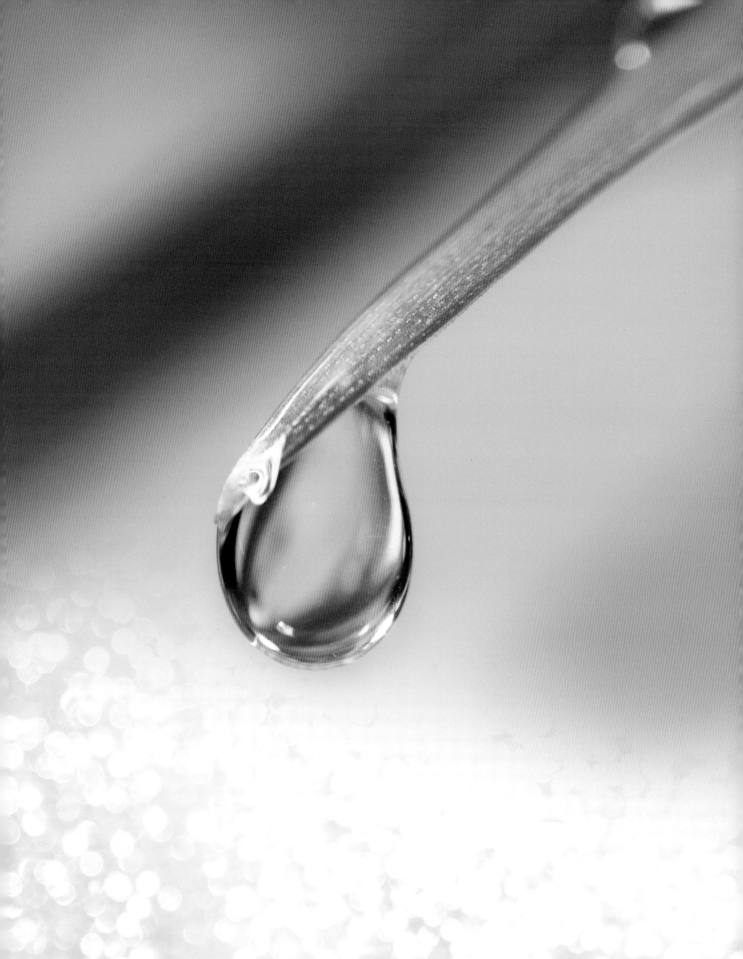

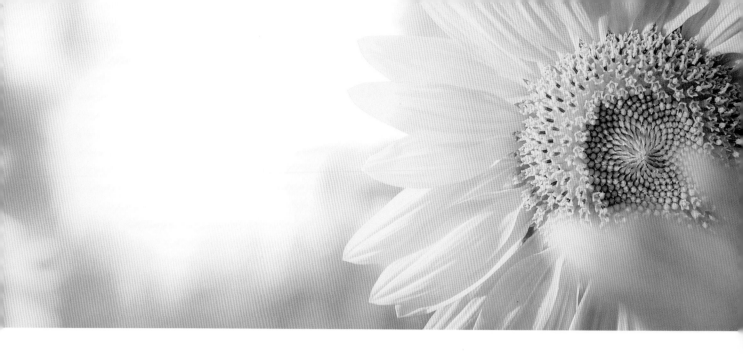

Sunlight

Our bodies were made to interact with the outside world. One evidence of this is our need of sunlight for our health and survival. The moment our skin comes into contact with the sun, our bodies begin to produce an important hormone called vitamin D. This hormone has a variety of health benefits that go beyond strong bones and teeth. It has been linked to a reduction in the incidence of heart disease[208] and the prevention of diabetes and multiple sclerosis.[209] Sunlight, together with exercise, can also improve mood and help stave off depression by boosting serotonin levels.[210] Additionally, it is an important component to our sleep-wake cycle and promotes quality sleep.[211]

Sunlight and Cancer

A number of studies have highlighted the importance of adequate sunlight in cancer prevention. Some of these studies have found that:

- Individuals who live at higher altitudes and, as a result, have reduced exposure to sunlight have a higher risk of both colon and breast cancer than those living in lower, sunlight-abundant altitudes.[212]
- A lack of UVB radiation from sunlight accounts for about 25 percent of breast cancer mortality rates.[213]

While the benefits of sunlight in health and cancer prevention are clear, overexposure increases the risk of skin cancer. So be sure to exercise caution when exposing yourself to the sun.

RECOMMENDATIONS:

- Aim for 15 minutes a day of sun exposure if you have a lighter skin tone. Those with a darker complexion should aim for 30 minutes a day.
- Sun exposure is safest in the morning before 10:00 A.M. or in the afternoon after 2:00 P.M.
- If you will be out in the sun for longer periods of time, use protective clothing like hats and long sleeves and keep yourself well hydrated.

Temperance

You have heard it before: everything in moderation. For the most part, this is true. After all, too much of even a good thing can be bad. Eat too much of the healthiest food and you will gain weight and experience many health problems. Sit too long in the sun and you will increase your risk of skin cancer. Drink too much water or get too much sleep, and you will disrupt normal body function and put yourself at risk. But if you want the best health possible, "everything in moderation" is just not enough. That's because while many things can be safely used in moderation, some things are best avoided altogether.

Research has demonstrated that smoking is damaging to health, promoting asthma and increasing cancer risk. Recreational drugs like marijuana, cocaine, and LSD have mood- and perception-altering qualities that are damaging to both physical and mental health. Alcohol consumption, even at low levels, increases cancer risk. Consumed at higher levels, it is implicated in everything from domestic abuse to car accidents.

Temperance is summed up in two important principles: moderately use the things that promote the health of body, mind, and spirit, and avoid things that are harmful. Because of this, it is best to avoid these substances altogether to enjoy maximum health.

> Temperance is summed up in two important principles: moderately use the things that promote the health of body, mind, and spirit, and avoid things that are harmful.

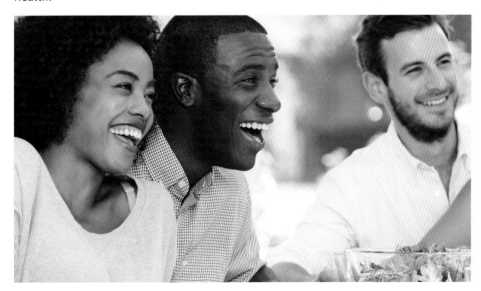

RECOMMENDATIONS:

- Be moderate and reasonable in diet, exercise, and other aspects of good health.
- Completely avoid substances and practices that compromise health, mental function, and positive social relationships. These include tobacco products, illicit drugs, and alcohol.

Did you know that adults breathe an average of 3,000 gallons of air every day? Air plays such a vital role in health that without it, we would die in minutes.[214] When we breathe out, we expel carbon dioxide, a waste product our bodies produce. When we breathe in, we take in oxygen, an element vital to cellular respiration, which is the process by which our bodies convert food into energy. Breathing fresh air helps

- clear the mind,
- relax the body,
- induce sound sleep, and
- reduce the risk of respiratory infections.

Just as the quality of the food we eat is important to good health, the quality of the air we breathe is also critically important. The World Health Organization estimates that worldwide, 7 million people die prematurely each year because of polluted air.[215] However, fresh air that is breathed in a natural environment provides many benefits for good health. For example, one study showed that walking in the forest, as compared to walking in the city, reduced blood pressure and controlled the stress hormone cortisol.[216]

Fresh Air and Cancer

Fresh air, particularly in a natural setting, has benefits when it comes to cancer prevention. Two studies showed that forest walks increased the levels of anticancer proteins in human participants. This benefit was not seen when subjects walked in cities.[217]

> Fresh air, particularly in a natural setting, has benefits when it comes to cancer prevention.

RECOMMENDATIONS:

- Breathe through your nose to protect your lungs from "unfiltered" air that may be cold, dry, or full of viruses and bacteria.
- Breathe from your abdomen by using your diaphragm to get the maximum benefit from each breath of air you take.
- Exercise outdoors whenever possible and seek natural surroundings.
- Go out for a breath of fresh air first thing in the morning.
- Throughout the day, take short breaks and go outside to get some fresh air.
- Keep your bedroom window open slightly when you sleep to let in fresh air.
- Avoid tight clothing and try to maintain good posture.

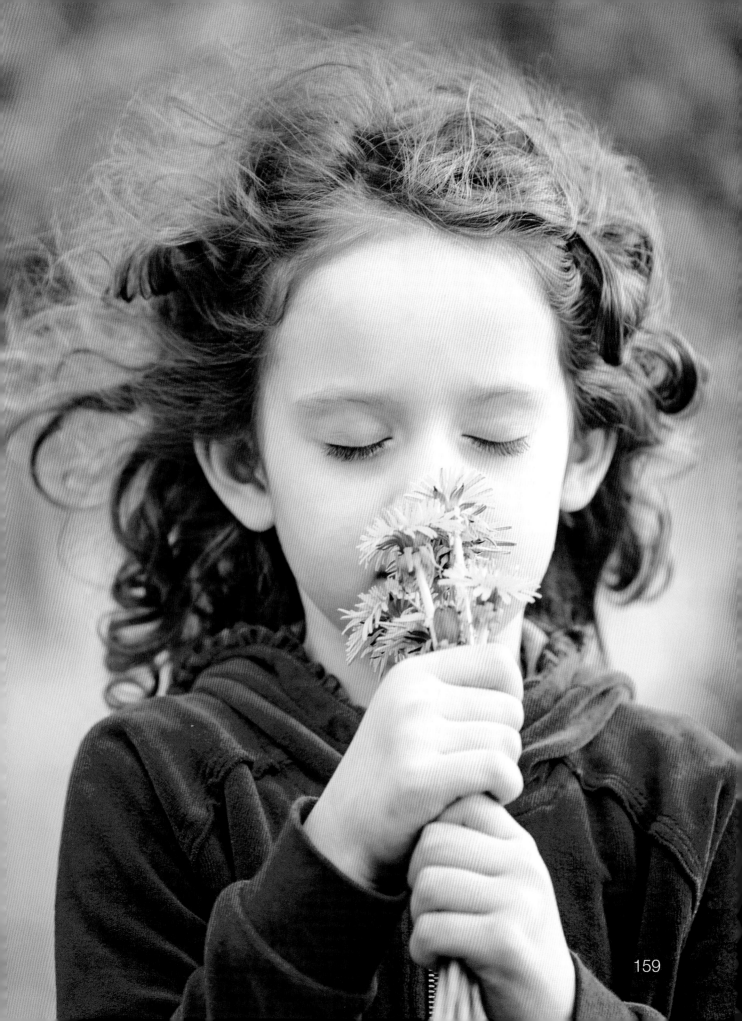

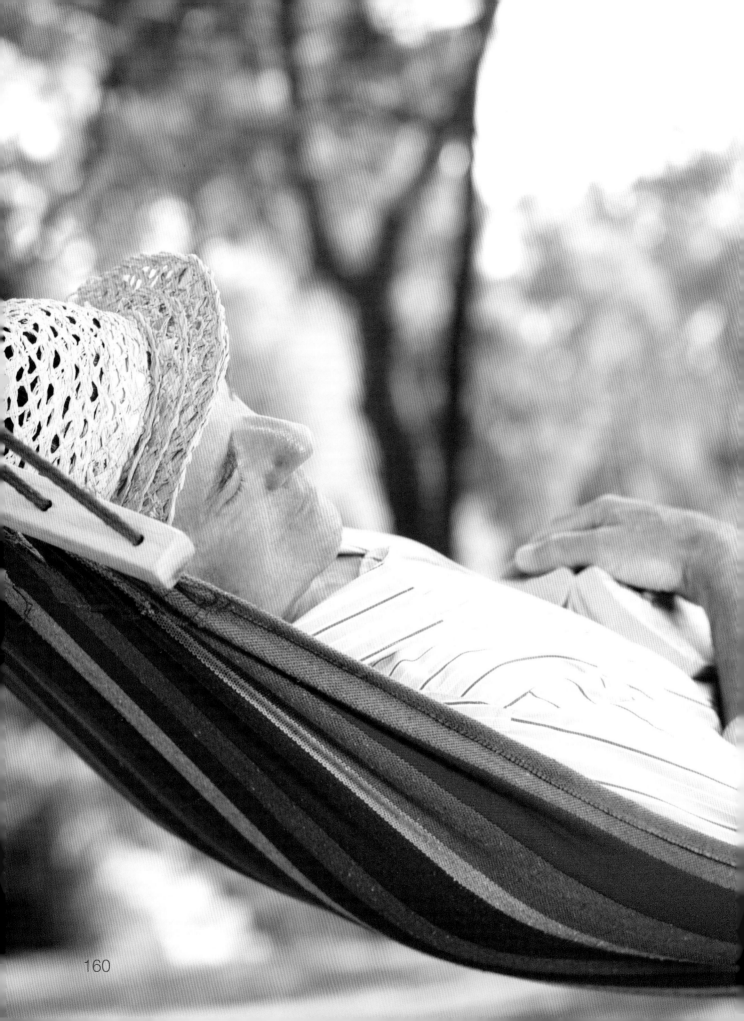

Rest

Sleep is not just for beauty. Rest in general (and sleep in particular) is critical to good overall health. In 2013, scientists learned that as we sleep, the brain clears out a neurotoxin called beta-amyloid at a faster rate than when we are awake.[218] This is significant because beta-amyloid is a toxin that accumulates in the brains of individuals with Alzheimer's disease. The "cleaning" function of sleep may contribute to sleep's ability to help us think more clearly and function at a higher level. But that isn't all:

- Sleep promotes normal growth in children and teenagers.
- Sleep facilitates the repair of heart and blood vessels.
- Sleep boosts the immune system.
- Sleep helps regulate hormones like insulin.[219]

Lack of sleep has been linked to depression, heart disease, diabetes, high blood pressure, stroke, and obesity.[220] It has even been linked to greater sensitivity to pain[221] and significantly increased risk of mortality.[222]

Sleep and Cancer

A number of studies have found a link between sleep disturbances and increased cancer risk:

- Women who are awake during the period of night when melatonin production is at its peak have higher incidences of breast cancer, as do graveyard shift workers and women who sleep in bright rooms.[223]
- Men who do rotating shift work are at a higher risk of developing prostate cancer.[224]
- Men who work at night are 1.76 times more likely to develop lung cancer, 2.03 times more likely to get colon cancer, and 1.74 times more likely to develop bladder cancer.[225]

Scientists believe sleep is connected with cancer risk because of a hormone called melatonin. Melatonin helps regulate our sleep-wake cycle and takes its cue from the sun. The body begins to secrete the hormone a couple of hours before bedtime, and at night melatonin levels peak and then level off as morning light approaches.

Melatonin *is highly sensitive to light*. Its production is *suppressed* by light, whether from the sun or from artificial sources, such as light bulbs, computers, and electronic devices. Melatonin suppression increases the release of estrogen by the ovaries, and increased estrogen is linked to increased breast cancer risk.[226] The mechanisms behind increased cancer risk for men who work night shifts are not clear. Scientists suspect that it, too, has to do with the suppression of melatonin levels.

RECOMMENDATIONS:

- Go to bed and wake up at the same time each day. Aim to sleep at least 7–8 hours per night.
- Go to bed at least a couple of hours before midnight for the best-quality sleep.
- Avoid electronic devices like TV, cell phones, and computers at least two hours before bed. The light these devices emit disrupts the secretion of melatonin.
- If you eat supper, make it light and eat early in the evening.
- Exercise daily to improve sleep quality.

Trust

It is easy to dismiss concepts such as trust and faith as irrelevant to health and well-being. Increasingly, however, scientists are discovering that these play an undeniable role in disease prevention and recovery.

- Individuals who regularly attend religious services have lower mortality rates than those who do not.[227]

- People with end-stage liver disease who are classified as "seeking God's help, having faith in God, trusting in God, and trying to discern God's will even in the disease" have improved survival rates.[228]

- Brain scans of people praying and meditating reveal physical changes in brain activity during times of prayer and meditation.[229] These changes may be linked to the improved health outcomes, such as lower stress and blood pressure, often associated with praying.[230]

For participants of addiction relief organizations like Alcoholics Anonymous and Narcotics Anonymous, trust in a "higher power" is a hallmark of the 12-Step recovery program.[231] But why turn outward to deal with problems that seem internal?

There's a saying that goes, "A joyful heart is good medicine, but a broken spirit dries up the bones."[232] This is because there is an undeniable connection between the state of the mind and the health of the body. Indeed, at the root of many physical and mental ailments may be a heart that is burdened with anxiety and guilt. But those who look to help outside of themselves find in a Higher Power reconciliation for the guilt of the past, strength to meet the challenges of the present, and hope and purpose for their future.

I don't know what your experience with faith has been. Sadly, the face of religion has been too often marred by the failings of imperfect people. Yet many who have chosen to look past the negativity have discovered something unexpected, beautiful, and liberating. They have found the very thing their souls were seeking.

The next page features additional resources for those who are interested in taking a closer look. From the question of suffering to the problem of addictions, you will find in these materials information to challenge and inspire; information that will help you experience health of body, mind, and soul.

> Those who maintain trust in a higher power experience many health benefits overall.

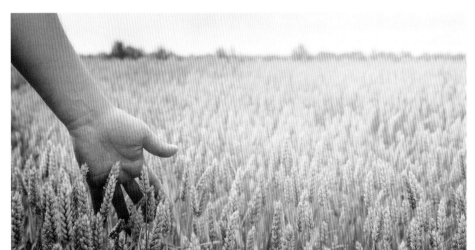

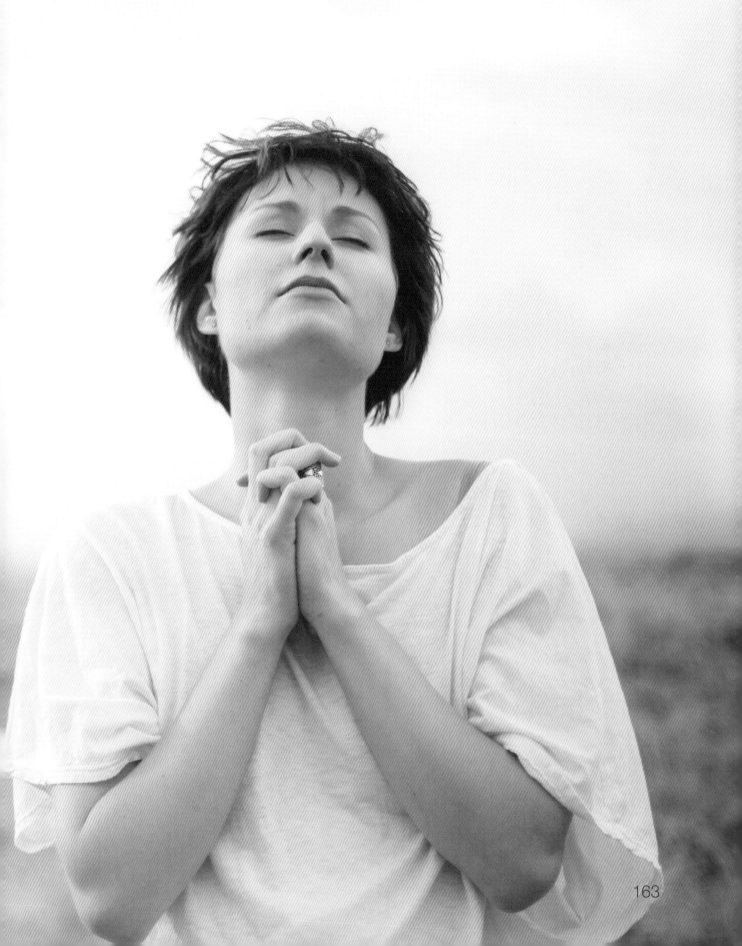

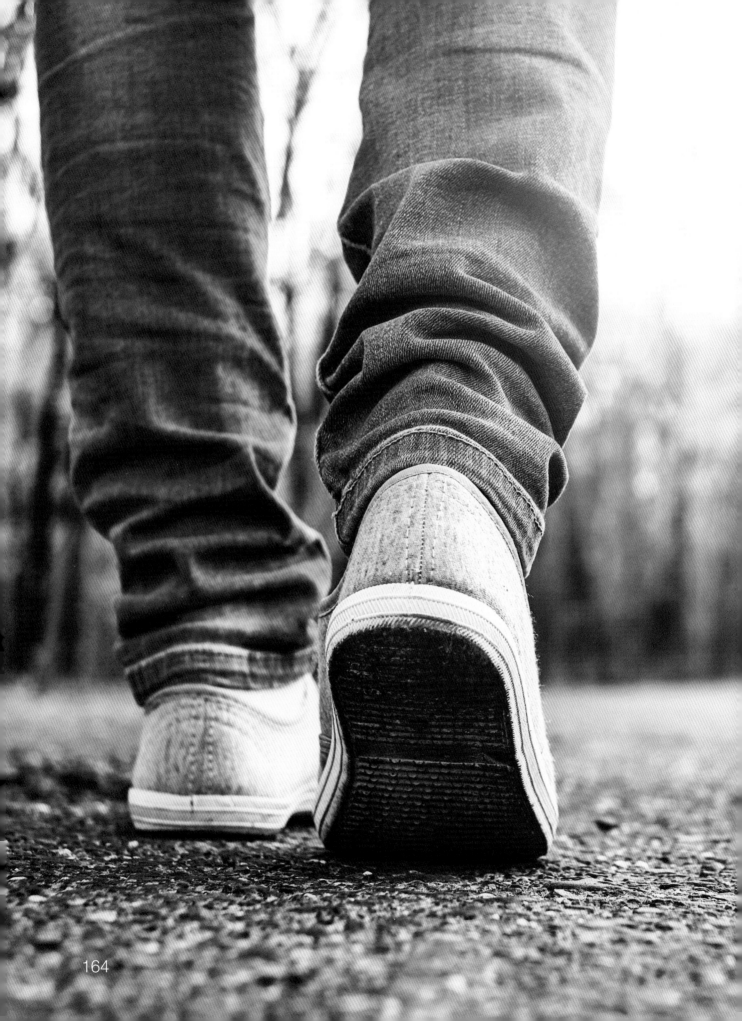

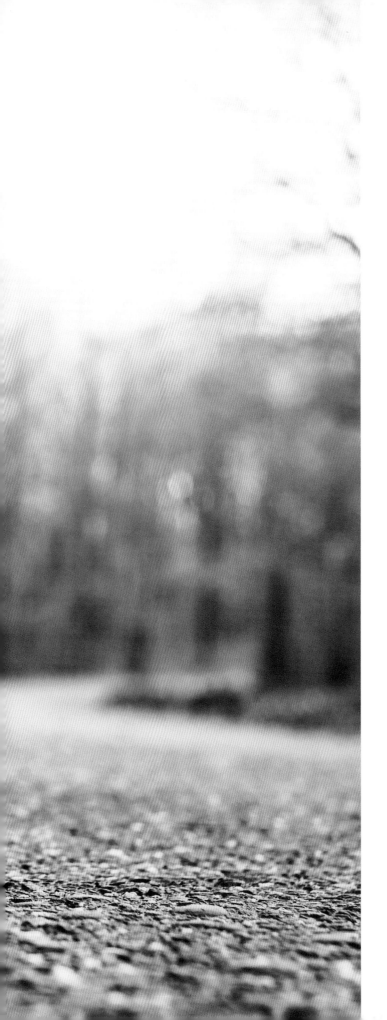

Your Turn

We have spent some time learning about the eight laws that help contribute to good health. Now, it is time to go from theory to practice. On the next page you will find a health assessment that will give you a snapshot view of your personal health. Are there areas in which you are doing well? Are there areas in which you can improve? Sometimes the first step on the journey to health is to figure out just where you are along the road. Once you have done that, then you can figure out where you want to go.

Step 1. How Healthy Is Your Lifestyle?

SCORE

1.	**Physical Activity** **30+ minutes of vigorous physical activity**	Little or no regular physical activity □0	2–3 days/week □5	4+ days/week □10	
2.	**Sleep** **Average hours per night**	Less than 6 hours per night □0	At least 7 hours per night and usually feel rested □5	7–8+ hours per night and always feel rested □10	
3.	**Fruits and Vegetables** **Servings per day** **(1 serving = 1 medium fruit or ½ cup cooked)**	0–2 servings per day □0	5–6 servings per day □5	7+ servings per day □10	
4.	**Whole Grains** **Breads and cereals**	Eat mostly white bread and refined cereals □0	Eat about half refined and half whole grains □5	Eat mostly whole-grain breads and cereals □10	
5.	**Animal Fat/High-Cholesterol Foods**	Regularly eat high-fat meats and dairy products □0	Eat only low-fat meats and dairy products □5	Seldom or never eat meat or dairy products □10	
6.	**Social Support and Interaction**	• I don't feel that I can count on help from family/friends if needed • Very little contact with them □0	• I have some support from family/friends if needed • I make occasional contact □5	• I have very good support from family/friends • I am always in contact with them □10	
7.	**Body Weight**	20+ excess pounds □0	10–15 pounds overweight or underweight □5	Very close to my ideal weight □10	
8.	**Blood Pressure**	140/90+ □0	120/80 to 139/89 □5	Less than 120/80 □10	
9.	**Breakfast**	Seldom eat breakfast □0	Eat breakfast most of the time □5	Eat a good breakfast every day □10	
10.	**Happiness**	• Not very happy or satisfied • Feel depressed at times □0	Pretty happy and satisfied □5	Very happy and satisfied with my life □10	
11.	**Time Outdoors**	Less than 15 minutes per day □0	15–45 minutes per day □5	Over one hour per day □10	
12.	**Spiritual Connection**	• Unsure of or have no spiritual or religious beliefs • Seldom or never participate in spiritual/religious groups □0	• Learning to have faith • Developing spiritual values • Meet occasionally with others of similar beliefs □5	• Have faith • Life is directed by spiritual values • Meet regularly with others of similar beliefs □10	
13.	**Water**	Drink less than 6 cups per day □0	Drink around 7 cups per day □5	Drink 8+ cups per day □10	

Total Healthy Lifestyle Score. Subtract 25 points if you are a smoker and/or drink alcohol more than once a day

0–45	50–85	90–115	120–130
VERY HIGH RISK	**INCREASED RISK**	**GOOD**	**EXCELLENT**

DISCLAIMER: By completing this assessment, I understand that all information and results I see is for general informational purposes only and is not intended to replace medical advice or treatment. I agree that I will take no action or inaction based solely on a product or suggestions made. I understand that lifestyle changes and/or questions about my health should be addressed directly to my licensed health provider.

Step 2. Personal Goals

Place a check mark next to the following lifestyle practices you would like to begin in order to improve your health.

- [ ] Eat 7+ servings of fruits and vegetables per day
- [ ] Eat a good daily breakfast and eat mostly whole grains
- [ ] Limit intake of animal fats and high-cholesterol foods
- [ ] Avoid alcoholic beverages
- [ ] Get 30+ minutes of intense physical activity at least 3 times per week

- [ ] Achieve and maintain a healthy weight
- [ ] Stop smoking
- [ ] Spend at least 45 minutes per day outdoors
- [ ] Get at least 7–8 hours of sleep per night and take time to relax
- [ ] Reconcile with friends and family and nurture supportive relationships

Step 3. My Commitment

It is my intent to improve my health by seeking to implement the changes listed above. Since studies show that it takes around twenty-one days to establish a habit, I commit to take the necessary steps to achieve better health and healing within the next three weeks.

Name _____

These important concepts, when internalized, will do more to improve your health and extend your life than all the technological wonders of modern medicine.

—Caldwell Esselstyn, MD

Endnotes

1. C. Staiger, "Comfrey: A Clinical Overview," *Phytotherapy Research* 26, no. 10, (2012), 1441–1448. https://doi.org/10.1002/ptr.4612.

2. This quote from Norman has been edited. The following is the unedited text: "Hi Afia, I know you could be busy but can't wait to tell you. My Lugs, my Abdominal, my Bladder are completely clear. They only find swollen in my lower throat/suffocate. They don't know where the Lymphoma cells gana. They cancel my chemotherapy treatment for now to do farther test to find out where the Lymphona cells was found by the biopsy fid go. Praise God. Praise God. Praise God. I got new life."

3. "Cancer Statistics at a Glance," Cancer Information, Canadian Cancer Society, accessed September 12, 2019, http://www.cancer.ca/en/cancer-information/cancer-101/cancer-statistics-at-a-glance/?region=on.

4. "Lifetime Risk of Developing or Dying From Cancer," Cancer A–Z, American Cancer Society, accessed September 12, 2019, http://www.cancer.org/cancer/cancerbasics/lifetime-probability-of-developing-or-dying-from-cancer.

5. D. W. Kufe et al., eds., "Multistage Carcinogenesis," *Holland-Frei Cancer Medicine*, 6th ed. (Hamilton, ON: BC Decker, 2003). Retrieved from http://www.ncbi.nlm.nih.gov/books/NBK13982/.

6. P. Anand et al., "Cancer Is a Preventable Disease That Requires Major Lifestyle Changes," *Pharmaceutical Research* 25, no. 9, (September 2008), 2097–2116, https://doi.org/10.1007/s11095-008-9661-9.

7. "The Adventist Health Study: Findings for Cancer," Findings for Past Studies, Adventist Health Study—1, School of Public Health, Loma Linda University, accessed September 12, 2019, http://publichealth.llu.edu/adventist-health-studies/findings/findings-past-studies/adventist-health-study-findings-cancer.

8. "Berries Seem to Burst With Cancer Protection," *American Institute for Cancer Research Newsletter*, April 15, 2013, http://www.aicr.org/publications/newsletter/2013-spring-119/berries-seem-to-burst-with-cancer-prevention.html?referrer=https://www.google.ca/.

9. N. P. Seeram, "Berry Fruits for Cancer Prevention: Current Status and Future Prospects," *Journal of Agricultural and Food Chemistry* 56, no. 3, (2008), 630–635. https://doi.org/10.1021/jf072504n.

10. Seeram, "Berry Fruits for Cancer Prevention: Current Status and Future Prospects," 630–635.

11. "How Fiber Helps Protect Against Cancer," Fiber, Physicians Committee for Responsible Medicine, accessed September 12, 2019, https://www.pcrm.org/health/cancer-resources/diet-cancer/nutrition/how-fiber-helps-protect-against-cancer.

12. G. D. Stoner et al., "Cancer Prevention With Freeze-Dried Berries and Berry Components," *Seminars in Cancer Biology* 17, no. 5, October 2007, 403–410, https://doi.org/10.1016/j.semcancer.2007.05.001.

13. C. Gerhauser, "Cancer Chemopreventive Potential of Apples, Apple Juice, and Apple Components," *Planta Medica* 74, no. 13, (October 2008), 1608–1624, https://doi.org/10.1055/s-0028-1088300.

14. Gerhauser, "Cancer Chemopreventive Potential of Apples, Apple Juice, and Apple Components," 1608–1624.

15. Gerhauser, 1608–1624.

16. D. A. Hyson, "A Comprehensive Review of Apples and Apple Components and Their Relationship to Human Health," *Advances in Nutrition: An International Review Journal* 2, no. 5, (September 2011), 408–420, https://doi.org/10.3945/an.111.000513.

17. J. Boyer and R. H. Liu, "Apple Phytochemicals and Their Health Benefits," *Nutrition Journal* 3, no. 5, (May 12, 2004), 12, https://doi.org/10.1186/1475-2891-3-5.

18. S. Gallus et al., "Does an Apple a Day Keep the Oncologist Away?" *Annals of Oncology* 16, no. 11, (November 2005), 1841–1844, https://doi.org/10.1093/annonc/mdi361.

19. "Apples," AICR's Foods That Fight Cancer™, American Institute for Cancer Research, accessed September 12, 2019, http://www.aicr.org/foods-that-fight-cancer/apples.html#research.

20. M. Matti, "Dirty Dozen List: Apples Top 2014 List of Most Pesticide-Contaminated Produce," CTV News, April 30, 2014, Health, http://www.ctvnews.ca/health/dirty-dozen-list-apples-top-2014-list-of-most-pesticide-contaminated-produce-1.1799569.

21. A. Nkondjock et al., "Dietary Intake of Lycopene Is Associated With Reduced Pancreatic Cancer Risk," *Journal of Nutrition* 135, no. 3, (March 1, 2005), 592–597, https://doi.org/10.1093/jn/135.3.592.

22. J. Higdon et al., "Carotenoids," Micronutrient Information Center, Linus Pauling Institute, Oregon State University, accessed September 12, 2019, http://lpi.oregonstate.edu/infocenter/phytochemicals/carotenoids/.

23. C. N. Holick et al., "Dietary Carotenoids, Serum β-Carotene, and Retinol and Risk of Lung Cancer in the Alpha-Tocopherol, Beta-Carotene Cohort Study," *American Journal of Epidemiology* 156, no. 6, (September 2002), 536–547, https://doi.org/10.1093/aje/kwf072.

24. K. Spector, "Raw Veggies Pack a Punch, But Cooking Can Unlock Key Benefits," cleveland.com, August 3, 2010,

Health and Fitness, http://www.cleveland.com/healthfit/index.ssf/2010/08/raw_veggies_can_pack_a_punch_b.html.

25. K. Zhou, and J. J. Raffoul, "Potential Anticancer Properties of Grape Antioxidants," *Journal of Oncology* 2012, no. 5, (2012), 803294, https://doi.org/10.1155/2012/803294.

26. A. Bishayee, "Cancer Prevention and Treatment With Resveratrol: From Rodent Studies to Clinical Trials," *Cancer Prevention Research* 2, no. 5, (May 2009), 409–418, https://doi.org/10.1158/1940-6207.CAPR-08-0160.

27. Bishayee, "Cancer Prevention and Treatment With Resveratrol," 409–418.

28. Zhou and Raffoul, "Potential Anticancer Properties of Grape Antioxidants," 803294.

29. Matti, "Dirty Dozen List."

30. N. D. Kim et al., "Chemopreventive and Adjuvant Therapeutic Potential of Pomegranate (*Punica granatum*) for Human Breast Cancer," *Breast Cancer Research and Treatment* 71, no. 3, (February 2002), 203–217, https://doi.org/10.1023/A:1014405730585.

31. A. J. Pantuck et al., "Phase II Study of Pomegranate Juice for Men With Rising Prostate-Specific Antigen Following Surgery or Radiation for Prostate Cancer," *Clinical Cancer Research* 12, no. 13, (July 2006), 4018–4026, https://doi.org/10.1158/1078-0432.CCR-05-2290.

32. J. A. Vinson et al., "Dried Fruits: Excellent *in Vitro* and *in Vivo* Antioxidants," *Journal of the American College of Nutrition* 24, no. 1, (2005), 44–50, https://doi.org/10.1080/07315724.2005.10719442.

33. D. Del Rio et al., "Dietary (Poly) Phenolics in Human Health: Structures, Bioavailability, and Evidence of Protective Effects Against Chronic Diseases," *Antioxidants and Redox Signaling* 18, no. 14, (April 4, 2013), 1818–1892, https://doi.org/10.1089/ars.2012.4581.

34. J. A. Vinson et al., "Dried Fruits: Excellent *in Vitro* and *in Vivo* Antioxidants," *Journal of the American College of Nutrition* 24, no. 1, (2005), 44–50, https://doi.org/10.1080/07315724.2005.10719442.

35. "The Adventist Health Study: Findings for Cancer."

36. "The Adventist Health Study: Findings for Cancer."

37. Matti, "Dirty Dozen List."

38. O. Oyebode et al., "Fruit and Vegetable Consumption and All-Cause, Cancer and CVD Mortality: Analysis of Health Survey for England Data," *Journal of Epidemiology and Community Health* 68, no. 9 (March 31, 2014), 856–852, https://doi.org/10.1136/jech-2013-203500.

39. Oyebode et al., "Fruit and Vegetable Consumption," 856–852.

40. A. Sifferlin, "Eat This Now: Rainbow Carrots," *Time*, August 20, 2013, Food and Drink, http://healthland.time.com/2013/08/20/eat-this-now-rainbow-carrots/.

41. M. P. Longnecker et al., "Intake of Carrots, Spinach, and Supplements Containing Vitamin A in Relation to Risk of Breast Cancer," *Cancer Epidemiology Biomarkers and Prevention* 6, no. 11, (November 1997), 887–892, https://cebp.aacrjournals.org/content/6/11/887.long.

42. P. Pisani et al., "Carrots, Green Vegetables and Lung Cancer: A Case-Control Study," *International Journal of Epidemiology* 15, no. 4, (December 1, 1986), 463–468, https://doi.org/10.1093/ije/15.4.463.

43. A. C. Butalla et al., "Effects of a Carrot Juice Intervention on Plasma Carotenoids, Oxidative Stress, and Inflammation in Overweight Breast Cancer Survivors," *Nutrition and Cancer* 64, no. 2, (2012), 331–341, https://doi.org/10.1080/01635581.2012.650779.

44. Y. Okuyama et al., "Inverse Associations Between Serum Concentrations of Zeaxanthin and Other Carotenoids and Colorectal Neoplasm in Japanese," *International Journal of Clinical Oncology* 19, no. 1, (February 2014), 87–97, https://doi.org/10.1007/s10147-013-0520-2.

45. R. Zaini, M. R. Clench, and C. L. Le Maitre, "Bioactive Chemicals From Carrot (*Daucus carota*) Juice Extracts for the Treatment of Leukemia," *Journal of Medicinal Food* 14, no. 11, (November 4, 2011), 1303–1312, https://doi.org/10.1089/jmf.2010.0284.

46. K. Wu et al., "Plasma and Dietary Carotenoids, and the Risk of Prostate Cancer: A Nested Case-Control Study," *Cancer Epidemiology Biomarkers and Prevention* 13, no. 2, (February 1, 2004), 260–269, https://doi.org/10.1158/1055-9965.EPI-03-0012.

47. University of Newcastle Upon Tyne, "Carrot Component Reduces Cancer Risk," ScienceDaily, February 18, 2005, https://www.sciencedaily.com/releases/2005/02/050212184702.htm.

48. S. T. Talcott, L. R. Howard, and C. H. Brenes, "Antioxidant Changes and Sensory Properties of Carrot Puree Processed With and Without Periderm Tissue," *Journal of Agricultural and Food Chemistry* 48, no. 4, (March 21, 2000), 1315–1321, https://doi.org/10.1021/jf9910178.

49. C. Miglio et al., "Effects of Different Cooking Methods on Nutritional and Physicochemical Characteristics of Selected Vegetables," *Journal of Agricultural and Food Chemistry* 56, no. 1, (December 11, 2007), 139–147, https://doi.org/10.1021/jf072304b.

50. C. Alasalvar et al., "Comparison of Volatiles, Phenolics, Sugars, Antioxidant Vitamins, and Sensory Quality of Different Colored Carrot Varieties," *Journal of Agricultural and Food Chemistry* 49, no. 3, (February 8, 2001), 1410–1416, https://doi.org/10.1021/jf000595h.

51. A. O. Jumaan et al., "Beta-Carotene Intake and Risk of Postmenopausal Breast Cancer," *Epidemiology* 10, no. 1, (January 1999), 49–53, https://www.ncbi.nlm.nih.gov/pubmed/9888279.

52. R. G. Ziegler, "A Review of Epidemiologic Evidence That Carotenoids Reduce the Risk of Cancer," *Journal of Nutrition* 119, no. 1, (January 1989), 116–122, https://doi

.org/10.1093/jn/119.1.116.

53. G. van Poppel and R. A. Goldbohm, "Epidemiologic Evidence for Beta-Carotene and Cancer Prevention," *American Journal of Clinical Nutrition* 62, no. 6, 1393S–1402S (December 1, 1995), https://doi.org/10.1093/ajcn/62.6.1393S.

54. M. A. Parasramka et al., "MicroRNA Profiling of Carcinogen-Induced Rat Colon Tumors and the Influence of Dietary Spinach," *Molecular Nutrition and Food Research* 56, no. 8, (May 29, 2012), 1259–1269, https://doi.org/10.1002/mnfr.201200117.

55. G. S. Omenn et al., "Effects of a Combination of Beta Carotene and Vitamin A on Lung Cancer and Cardiovascular Disease," *New England Journal of Medicine* 334, no. 18, (May 2, 1996), 1150–1155, https://doi.org/10.1056/NEJM199605023341802.

56. J. Czapski, "Cancer Preventing Properties of Cruciferous Vegetables," *Vegetable Crops Research Bulletin* 70, no. 1, (July 31, 2009), 5–18, https://doi.org/10.2478/v10032-009-0001-3.

57. Czapski, "Cancer Preventing Properties of Cruciferous Vegetables" 5–18.

58. Czapski, 5–18.

59. M. K. Shea et al., "Vitamin K and Vitamin D Status: Associations With Inflammatory Markers in the Framingham Offspring Study," *American Journal of Epidemiology* 167, no. 3, (February 2008), 313–320, https://doi.org/10.1093/aje/kwm306.

60. M. J. Shearer and P. Newman, "Metabolism and Cell Biology of Vitamin K," *Thrombosis and Haemostasis* 100, no. 4, (2008), 530–547, https://doi.org/10.1160/TH08-03-0147.

61. "Eating Healthy With Cruciferous Vegetables," The World's Healthiest Foods, The George Mateljan Foundation, accessed September 12, 2019, http://www.whfoods.com/genpage.php?tname=btnewsanddbid=126.

62. P. Gonçalves and F. Martel, "Butyrate and Colorectal Cancer: The Role of Butyrate Transport," *Current Drug Metabolism* 14, no. 9, (2013), 994–1008, https://doi.org/10.2174/1389200211314090006.

63. L. Li et al., "Cruciferous Vegetable Consumption and the Risk of Pancreatic Cancer: A Meta-Analysis," *World Journal of Surgical Oncology* 13, no. 1, (2015), 44, https://doi.org/10.1186/s12957-015-0454-4.

64. V. A. Kirsh et al., "Prospective Study of Fruit and Vegetable Intake and Risk of Prostate Cancer," *Journal of the National Cancer Institute* 99, no. 15, (August 2007), 1200–1209, https://doi.org/10.1093/jnci/djm065.

65. E. L. Richman, P. R. Carroll, and J. M. Chan, "Vegetable and Fruit Intake After Diagnosis and Risk of Prostate Cancer Progression," *International Journal of Cancer* 131, no. 1, (August 5, 2011), 201–210, https://doi.org/10.1002/ijc.26348.

66. L. Tang et al., "Cruciferous Vegetable Intake Is Inversely Associated With Lung Cancer Risk Among Smokers: A Case-Control Study," *BMC Cancer* 10, no. 1, (April 27, 2010), 162,

67. C. Cerella et al., "Chemical Properties and Mechanisms Determining the Anti-Cancer Action of Garlic-Derived Organic Sulfur Compounds," *Anti-Cancer Agents in Medicinal Chemistry* (Formerly *Current Medicinal Chemistry—Anti-Cancer Agents*) 11, no. 3, (2011), 267–271, https://doi.org/10.2174/187152011795347522.

68. F. Khanum, K. R. Anilakumar, and K. R. Viswanathan, "Anticarcinogenic Properties of Garlic: A Review," *Critical Reviews in Food Science and Nutrition* 44, no. 6, (2004), 479–488, https://doi.org/10.1080/10408690490886700.

69. Khanum, Anilakumar, and Viswanathan, "Anticarcinogenic Properties of Garlic," 479–488.

70. K. A. Steinmetz et al., "Vegetables, Fruit, and Colon Cancer in the Iowa Women's Health Study," *American Journal of Epidemiology* 139, no. 1, (January 1994), 1–15, https://doi.org/10.1093/oxfordjournals.aje.a116921.

71. A. W. Hsing et al., "Allium Vegetables and Risk of Prostate Cancer: A Population-Based Study," *Journal of the National Cancer Institute* 94, no. 21, (November 6, 2002), 1648–1651, https://doi.org/10.1093/jnci/94.21.1648.

72. "Garlic and Cancer Prevention," accessed January 25, 2016, http://www.cancer.gov/cancertopics/factsheet/prevention/garlic-and-cancer-prevention#r11; J. M. Chan, F. Wang, and E. A. Holly, "Vegetable and Fruit Intake and Pancreatic Cancer in a Population-Based Case-Control Study in the San Francisco Bay Area," *Cancer Epidemiology Biomarkers and Prevention* 14, no. 9, (September 2005), 2093–2097, https://doi.org/10.1158/1055-9965.EPI-05-0226.

73. "Eating Raw Garlic Can Prevent Cancer, Study Suggests," CBC News, August 07, 2013, accessed September 12, 2019, http://www.cbc.ca/news/health/eating-raw-garlic-can-prevent-cancer-study-suggests-1.1343422; Z. Y. Jin et al., "Raw Garlic Consumption as a Protective Factor for Lung Cancer, a Population-Based Case-Control Study in a Chinese Population," *Cancer Prevention Research* 6, no. 7, (July 2013), 711–718, https://doi.org/10.1158/1940-6207.CAPR-13-0015.

74. J. A. Milner, "Garlic: Its Anticarcinogenic and Antitumorigenic Properties," *Nutrition Reviews* 54, no. 11, (November 1, 1996), S82–S86, https://doi.org/10.1111/j.1753-4887.1996.tb03823.x.

75. S. S. Lang, "Onion a Day Keeps Doctor Away? Cornell Researchers Find Some Onions Do Indeed Have Excellent Anti-Cancer Benefits," *Cornell Chronicle*, October 7, 2004, http://www.news.cornell.edu/stories/2004/10/some-onions-have-excellent-anti-cancer-benefits.

76. J. Slavin, "Why Whole Grains Are Protective: Biological Mechanisms," *Proceedings of the Nutrition Society* 62, no. 1, (February 2003), 129–134, https://doi.org/10.1079/PNS2002221.

77. Slavin, "Why Whole Grains Are Protective," 129–134.

78. L. U. Thompson, "Antioxidants and Hormone-Mediated

Health Benefits of Whole Grains," *Critical Reviews in Food Science and Nutrition* 34, no. 5–6, (1994), 473–497, https://doi.org/10.1080/10408399409527676.

79. J. Slavin, D. Jacobs, and L. Marquart, "Whole-Grain Consumption and Chronic Disease: Protective Mechanisms," *Nutrition and Cancer* 27, no. 1, (1997), 14–21, https://doi.org/10.1080/01635589709514495.

80. "Whole Wheat," The World's Healthiest Foods, The George Mateljan Foundation, accessed September 13, 2019, http://www.whfoods.com/genpage.php?tname=foodspice&dbid=66.

81. J. Y. Dong et al., "Dietary Fiber Intake and Risk of Breast Cancer: A Meta-Analysis of Prospective Cohort Studies," *American Journal of Clinical Nutrition* 94, no. 3, (September 2011), 900–905, https://doi.org/10.3945/ajcn.111.015578.

82. D. Aune et al., "Dietary Fibre, Whole Grains, and Risk of Colorectal Cancer: Systematic Review and Dose-Response Meta-Analysis of Prospective Studies," *BMJ* 343, (November 10, 2011), https://doi.org/10.1136/bmj.d6617.

83. J. R. Hebert et al., "Nutritional and Socioeconomic Factors in Relation to Prostate Cancer Mortality: A Cross-National Study," *Journal of the National Cancer Institute* 90, no. 21, (November 4, 1998), 1637–1647, https://doi.org/10.1093/jnci/90.21.1637.

84. "The Adventist Health Study: Findings for Cancer."

85. "The Adventist Health Study: Findings for Cancer."

86. P. P. Bao et al., "Fruit, Vegetable, and Animal Food Intake and Breast Cancer Risk by Hormone Receptor Status," *Nutrition and Cancer* 64, no. 6, (August 3, 2012), 806–819, https://doi.org/10.1080/01635581.2012.707277.

87. C. A. Adebamowo et al., "Dietary Flavonols and Flavonol-Rich Foods Intake and the Risk of Breast Cancer," *International Journal of Cancer* 114, no. 4, (April 20, 2005), 628–633, https://doi.org/10.1002/ijc.20741.

88. L. N. Kolonel et al., "Vegetables, Fruits, Legumes and Prostate Cancer: A Multiethnic Case-Control Study," *Cancer Epidemiology Biomarkers and Prevention* 9, no. 8, (August 2000), 795–804, https://cebp.aacrjournals.org/content/9/8/795.long.

89. M. McCullough, "The Bottom Line on Soy and Breast Cancer Risk," *Expert Voices Blog—Timely Insights on Cancer Topics From the Experts of the American Cancer Society,* August 2, 2012, http://blogs.cancer.org/expertvoices/2012/08/02/the-bottom-line-on-soy-and-breast-cancer-risk/.

90. A. H. Wu et al., "Soy Intake and Breast Cancer Risk in Singapore Chinese Health Study," *British Journal of ancer* 99, no. 1, (July 8, 2008), 196–200, https://doi.org/10.1038/sj.bjc.6604448.

91. Kolonel et al., "Vegetables, Fruits, Legumes and Prostate Cancer," 795–804.

92. M. M. Lee et al., "Soy and Isoflavone Consumption in Relation to Prostate Cancer Risk in China," *Cancer Epidemiology Biomarkers and Prevention* 12, no. 7, (July 2003), 665–668, https://cebp.aacrjournals.org/content/12/7/665.long.

93. B. K. Jacobsen, S. F. Knutsen, and G. E. Fraser, "Does High Soy Milk Intake Reduce Prostate Cancer Incidence? The Adventist Health Study (United States)," *Cancer Causes and Control* 9, no. 6, (December 1998), 553–557, https://doi.org/10.1023/A:1008819500080.

94. "Worldwide Cancer Incidence Statistics," Cancer Research UK, accessed January 25, 2016, http://www.cancerresearchuk.org/health-professional/cancer-statistics/worldwide-cancer/incidence#heading-Zero.

95. Cancer Research UK, "Worldwide Cancer Incidence Statistics."

96. Cancer Research UK, "Worldwide Cancer Incidence Statistics."

97. C. Fuchs, "Large Study Links Nut Consumption to Reduced Death Rate," Nutrition & Diet, Dana-Farber Cancer Institute, November 20, 2013, http://www.dana-farber.org/Newsroom/News-Releases/Large-study-links-nut-consumption-to-reduced-death-rate.aspx.

98. Fuchs, "Large Study Links Nut Consumption to Reduced Death Rate."

99. C. Ip, and D. J. Lisk, "Bioactivity of Selenium From Brazil Nut for Cancer Prevention and Selenoenzyme Maintenance," *Nutrition and Cancer* 21, no. 3, (1994), 203–212, https://doi.org/10.1080/01635589409514319.

100. W. E. Hardman, "Walnuts Have Potential for Cancer Prevention and Treatment in Mice," *Journal of Nutrition* 144, no. 4, (February 5, 2014), 555S–560S, https://doi.org/10.3945/jn.113.188466.

101. R. J. Reiter et al., "A Walnut-Enriched Diet Reduces the Growth of LNCaP Human Prostate Cancer Xenografts in Nude Mice," *Cancer Investigation* 31, no. 6, (June 11, 2013), 365–373, https://doi.org/10.3109/07357907.2013.800095.

102. Hardman, "Walnuts Have Potential for Cancer Prevention and Treatment in Mice," 555S–560S.

103. J. Higdon and V. Drake, "Lignans," Micronutrient Information Center, Linus Pauling Institute, Oregon State University, accessed September 13, 2019, http://lpi.oregonstate.edu/mic/dietary-factors/phytochemicals/lignans.

104. E. C. Lowcock, M. Cotterchio, and B. A. Boucher, "Consumption of Flaxseed, a Rich Source of Lignans, Is Associated With Reduced Breast Cancer Risk," *Cancer Causes and Control* 24, no. 4, (April 2013), 813–816, https://doi.org/10.1007/s10552-013-0155-7.

105. L. U. Thompson et al., "Dietary Flaxseed Alters Tumor Biological Markers in Postmenopausal Breast Cancer," *Clinical Cancer Research* 11, no. 10, (May 2005), 3828–3835, https://doi.org/10.1158/1078-0432.CCR-04-2326.

106. W. Demark-Wahnefried et al., "Flaxseed Supplementation (Not Dietary Fat Restriction) Reduces Prostate Cancer Proliferation Rates in Men Presurgery," *Cancer Epidemiology Biomarkers and Prevention* 17, no. 12, (December 2008), 3577–3587, https://doi.org/10.1158/1055-9965.EPI-08-0008.

107. M. Hedelin et al., "Dietary Phytoestrogen, Serum Enterolactone and Risk of Prostate Cancer: The Cancer Prostate Sweden Study (Sweden)," *Cancer Causes and Control* 17, no. 2, (March 2006), 169–180, https://doi.org/10.1007/s10552-005-0342-2.

108. L. Sun, C. Luo, and J. Liu, "Hydroxytyrosol Induces Apoptosis in Human Colon Cancer Cells Through ROS Generation," *Food and Function* 5, no. 8, (2014), 1909–1914, https://doi.org/10.1039/c4fo00187g.

109. L. Lucas, A. Russell, and R. Keast, "Molecular Mechanisms of Inflammation. Anti-Inflammatory Benefits of Virgin Olive Oil and the Phenolic Compound Oleocanthal," *Current Pharmaceutical Design* 17, no. 8, (2011), 754–768, https://doi.org/10.2174/138161211795428911.

110. A. Trichopoulou et al., "Cancer and Mediterranean Dietary Traditions," *Cancer Epidemiology Biomarkers and Prevention* 9, no. 9, (September 2000), 869–873, .

111. Universitat Autònoma de Barcelona, "Key Mechanism Links Virgin Olive Oil to Protection Against Breast Cancer" *ScienceDaily*, June 30, 2010, https://www.sciencedaily.com/releases/2010/06/100630115019.htm.

112. J. M. Martin-Moreno et al., "Dietary Fat, Olive Oil Intake and Breast Cancer Risk," *International Journal of Cancer* 58, no. 6, (September 15, 1994), 774–780, https://doi.org/10.1002/ijc.2910580604.

113. A. Trichopoulou et al., "Consumption of Olive Oil and Specific Food Groups in Relation to Breast Cancer Risk in Greece," *Journal of the National Cancer Institute* 87, no. 2, (January 18, 1995), 110–116, https://doi.org/10.1093/jnci/87.2.110.

114. M. Stoneham et al., "Olive Oil, Diet and Colorectal Cancer: An Ecological Study and a Hypothesis," *Journal of Epidemiology and Community Health* 54, no. 10, (October 1, 2000), 756–760, https://doi.org/10.1136/jech.54.10.756.

115. R. E. Kopec et al., "Avocado Consumption Enhances Human Postprandial Provitamin A Absorption and Conversion From a Novel High–β-carotene Tomato Sauce and From Carrots," *Journal of Nutrition* 144, no. 8, (August 2014), 1158–1166, https://doi.org/10.3945/jn.113.187674.

116. Q. Y. Lu et al., "Inhibition of Prostate Cancer Cell Growth by an Avocado Extract: Role of Lipid-Soluble Bioactive Substances," *Journal of Nutritional Biochemistry* 16, no. 1, (January 2005), 23–30, https://doi.org/10.1016/j.jnutbio.2004.08.003.

117. E. A. Lee et al., "Targeting Mitochondria With Avocatin B Induces Selective Leukemia Cell Death," *Cancer Research* 75, no. 12, (June 2015), 2478–2488, https://doi.org/10.1158/0008-5472.CAN-14-2676.

118. T. C. Campbell and T. M. Campbell II, "A House of Proteins," *The China Study: Startling Implications for Diet, Weight Loss and Long-Term Health* 36, (Dallas, Texas: BenBella Books, 2006), 36.

119. W. J. Cromie, "Growth Factor Raises Cancer Risk," *Harvard University Gazette*, April 2, 1999, http://news.harvard.edu/gazette/1999/04.22/igf1.story.html.

120. J. M. Chan et al., "Insulin-like Growth Factor-I (IGF-I) and IGF Binding Protein-3 as Predictors of Advanced-Stage Prostate Cancer," *Journal of the National Cancer Institute* 94, no. 14, (July 17, 2002), 1099–1106, https://doi.org/10.1093/jnci/94.14.1099.

121. S. Q. Doi et al., "Low-Protein Diet Suppresses Serum Insulin-Like Growth Factor-1 and Decelerates the Progression of Growth Hormone-Induced Glomerulosclerosis," *American Journal of Nephrology* 21, no. 4, (July–August, 2001), 331–339, https://doi.org/10.1159/000046270.

122. K. Skog et al., "Effect of Cooking Temperature on the Formation of Heterocyclic Amines in Fried Meat Products and Pan Residues," *Carcinogenesis* 16, no. 4, (April 1995), 861–867, https://doi.org/10.1093/carcin/16.4.861.

123. D. Buettner, "Longevity: The Secrets of Long Life," *National Geographic*, November 2005, http://ngm.nationalgeographic.com/2005/11/longevity-secrets/buettner-text.

124. M. G. Knize and J. S. Felton, "Formation and Human Risk of Carcinogenic Heterocyclic Amines Formed From Natural Precursors in Meat," *Nutrition Reviews* 63, no. 5, (May 2005), 158–165, https://doi.org/10.1111/j.1753-4887.2005.tb00133.x.

125. T. Sugimura et al., "Heterocyclic Amines: Mutagens/Carcinogens Produced During Cooking of Meat and Fish," *Cancer Science* 95, no. 4, (April 2004), 290–299, https://doi.org/10.1111/j.1349-7006.2004.tb03205.x.

126. D. H. Phillips, "Polycyclic Aromatic Hydrocarbons in the Diet," *Mutation Research/Genetic Toxicology and Environmental Mutagenesis* 443, nos. 1–2, (July 15, 1999), 139–147, https://doi.org/10.1016/S1383-5742(99)00016-2.

127. G. D. Pamplona-Roger, *Encyclopedia of Foods and Their Healing Power: A Guide to Food Science and Diet Therapy* vol. 1 (Madrid, Spain: Editorial Safelíz, 2001), 276.

128. Pamplona-Roger, *Encyclopedia of Foods and Their Healing Power*, 276.

129. A. Roeder, "Red Meat Consumption and Breast Cancer Risk," Harvard T. H. Chan School of Public Health, October 09, 2014, http://www.hsph.harvard.edu/news/features/red-meat-consumption-and-breast-cancer-risk/.

130. F. Lubin, Y. Wax, and B. Modan, "Role of Fat, Animal Protein, and Dietary Fiber in Breast Cancer Etiology: A Case-Control Study," *Journal of the National Cancer Institute* 77, no. 3, (September 1, 1986), 605–612, https://doi.org/10.1093/jnci/77.3.605.

131. E. M. John et al., "Meat Consumption, Cooking Practices, Meat Mutagens, and Risk of Prostate Cancer," *Nutrition and Cancer* 63, no. 4, (April 26, 2011), 525–537, https://doi.org/10.1080/01635581.2011.539311.

132. "Red Meat and Colon Cancer," Harvard Men's Health Watch, Harvard Health Publishing, Harvard Medical School, January 2008, http://www.health.harvard.edu/family_health _guide/red-meat-and-colon-cancer; S. Rohrmann et al., "Meat Consumption and Mortality—Results From the European Prospective Investigation Into Cancer and Nutrition," *BMC Medicine* 11, no. 1, (March 7, 2013), 63, https://doi .org/10.1186/1741-7015-11-63.

133. M. E. Levine et al., "Low Protein Intake Is Associated With a Major Reduction in IGF-1, Cancer, and Overall Mortality in the 65 and Younger but Not Older Population," *Cell Metabolism* 19, no. 3, (March 4, 2014), 407–417, https://doi .org/10.1016/j.cmet.2014.02.006.

134. "Red Meat and Colon Cancer."

135. "Red Meat and Colon Cancer."

136. Campbell and Campbell, *The China Study*, 54–59.

137. C. H. Kroenke et al., "High- and Low-Fat Dairy Intake, Recurrence, and Mortality After Breast Cancer Diagnosis," *Journal of the National Cancer Institute* 105, no. 9, (May 1, 2013), 616–623, https://doi.org/10.1093/jnci/djt027.

138. J. M. Chan et al., "Dairy Products, Calcium, Phosphorous, Vitamin D, and Risk of Prostate Cancer (Sweden)," *Cancer Causes and Control* 9, no. 6, (December 1998), 559–566, https://doi.org/10.1023/A:1008823601897.

139. A. H. Wu, M. C. Pike, and D. O. Stram, "Meta-Analysis: Dietary Fat Intake, Serum Estrogen Levels, and the Risk of Breast Cancer," *Journal of the National Cancer Institute* 91, no. 6, (March 17, 1999), 529–534, https://doi.org/10.1093 /jnci/91.6.529.

140. J. M. Chan and E. L. Giovannucci, "Dairy Products, Calcium, and Vitamin D and Risk of Prostate Cancer," *Epidemiologic Reviews* 23, no. 1, (March 1, 2001), 87–92, https://doi.org/10.1093/oxfordjournals.epirev.a000800.

141. J. M. Chan et al., "Dairy Products, Calcium, and Prostate Cancer Risk in the Physicians' Health Study," *American Journal of Clinical Nutrition* 74, no. 4, (October 1, 2001), 549–554, https://doi.org/10.1093/ajcn/74.4.549.

142. C. S. Spina et al., "Vitamin D and Cancer," *Anticancer Research* 26, no. 4A, (2006), 2515–2524, https://pdfs.semanticscholar. org/5ee1/84b34fa837e2f08deed02437449130050472.pdf.

143. H. Kesteloot, E. Lesaffre, and J. V. Joossens, "Dairy Fat, Saturated Animal Fat, and Cancer Risk," *Preventive Medicine* 20, no. 2, (March 1991), 226–236, https://doi.org/10.1016/0091 -7435(91)90022-V.

144. E. Cho et al., "Premenopausal Fat Intake and Risk of Breast Cancer," *Journal of the National Cancer Institute* 95, no. 14, (July 16, 2003), 1079–1085, https://doi.org/10.1093 /jnci/95.14.1079.

145. K. K. Carroll, "Experimental Evidence of Dietary Factors and Hormone-Dependent Cancers," *Cancer Research* 35, no. 11, (November 1975), 3374–3383, https://doi.org/10.1093

/jnci/95.14.1079.

146. Campbell and Campbell, *The China Study*," 60–62.

147. "Canadian Alcohol and Drug Use Monitoring Survey," Drug and Alcohol Use Statistics, Government of Canada, updated April 2, 2014, http://www.hc-sc.gc.ca/hc-ps/drugs -drogues/stat/_2011/summary-sommaire-eng.php.

148. "Alcohol Facts and Statistics," National Institute on Alcohol Abuse and Alcoholism, National Institutes of Health, updated August 2018, http://www.niaaa.nih.gov/alcohol -health/overview-alcohol-consumption/alcohol-facts-and -statistics.

149. V. Poznyak et al., *Global Status Report on Alcohol and Health—2014*, (Luxembourg World Health Organization, 2014), https://www.who.int/substance_abuse/publications /alcohol_2014/en/.

150. G. Pöschl and H. K. Seitz, "Alcohol and Cancer," *Alcohol and Alcoholism* 39, no. 3, (May 2004), 155–165, https://doi .org/10.1093/alcalc/agh057.

151. Pöschl and Seitz, "Alcohol and Cancer," 155–165.

152. C. M. Ulrich, "Folate and Cancer Prevention: A Closer Look at a Complex Picture," *American Journal of Clinical Nutrition* 86, no. 2, (August 1, 2007), 271–273, https://doi .org/10.1093/ajcn/86.2.271.

153. Pöschl and Seitz, "Alcohol and Cancer," 155–165.

154. T. J. Key, "Serum Oestradiol and Breast Cancer Risk," *Endocrine-Related Cancer* 6, no. 2, (June 1999), 175–180, https://doi.org/10.1677/erc.0.0060175.

155. V. Bagnardi et al., "Light Alcohol Drinking and Cancer: A Meta-Analysis," *Annals of Oncology* 24, no. 2, (February 2013), 301–308, https://doi.org/10.1093/annonc/mds337.

156. "Grapes and Grape Juice," Foods That Fight Cancer, American Institute for Cancer Research, accessed September 13, 2019, http://www.aicr.org/foods-that-fight -cancer/foodsthatfightcancer_grapes_and_grape_juice .html.

157. S. C. Larsson, L. Bergkvist, and A. Wolk, "Consumption of Sugar and Sugar-Sweetened Foods and the Risk of Pancreatic Cancer in a Prospective Study," *American Journal of Clinical Nutrition* 84, no. 5, (November 2006), 1171–1176, https://doi.org/10.1093/ajcn/84.5.1171.

158. M. L. Slattery et al., "Dietary Sugar and Colon Cancer," *Cancer Epidemiology Biomarkers and Prevention* 6, no. 9 (September 1997), 677–685, https://cebp.aacrjournals.org /content/6/9/677.long.

159. S. Seely and D. F. Horrobin, "Diet and Breast Cancer: the Possible Connection With Sugar Consumption," *Medical Hypotheses* 11, no. 3, (July 1983), 319–327, https://doi .org/10.1016/0306-9877(83)90095-6.

160. Larsson, Bergkvist, and Wolk, "Consumption of Sugar and Sugar-sweetened Foods," 1171–1176.

161. Larsson, Bergkvist, and Wolk, 1171–1176.

162. Seely and Horrobin, "Diet and Breast Cancer," 319–327.

163. M. Strnad, "Povećana konzumacija soli izaziva veći osjećaj žeđi, što povećava unos pića veće energetske vrijednosti i tako utječe na debljanje. Kada se radi o Menierovoj bolesti, pokazano je da prehrana s malo soli smanjuje učestalost i težinu [Salt and Cancer][Abstract]," *Acta Medica Croatica* 64, no. 2, (May 2010), 159–161, http://www.ncbi.nlm.nih.gov/pubmed/20649083.

164. S. Tsugane, "Salt, Salted Food Intake, and Risk of Gastric Cancer: Epidemiologic Evidence," *Cancer Science* 96, no. 1, (January 13, 2005), 1–6, https://doi.org/10.1111/j.1349 -7006.2005.00006.x.

165. X. Q. Wang, P. D. Terry, and H. Yan, "Review of Salt Consumption and Stomach Cancer Risk: Epidemiological and Biological Evidence," *World Journal of Gastroenterology* 15, no. 18, (March 14, 2009), 2204, https://doi.org/10.3748 /wjg.15.2204.

166. K. Shikata et al., "A Prospective Study of Dietary Salt Intake and Gastric Cancer Incidence in a Defined Japanese Population: The Hisayama Study," *International Journal of Cancer* 119, no. 1, (April 17, 2006), 196–201, https://doi .org/10.1002/ijc.21822.

167. R. Kumar Phukan et al., "Role of Dietary Habits in the Development of Esophageal Cancer in Assam, the North-Eastern Region of India," *Nutrition and Cancer* 39, no. 2, (2001), 204–209, https://doi.org/10.1207/S15327914nc392_7.

168. A. Mathew et al., "Diet and Stomach Cancer: A Case-Control Study in South India," *European Journal of Cancer Prevention* 9, no. 2, (April 2000), 89–98, https://insights.ovid .com/pubmed?pmid=10830575.

169. U. Kapil et al., "Assessment of Risk Factors in Laryngeal Cancer in India: A Case-Control Study," *Asian Pacific Journal of Cancer Prevention* 6, no. 2, (February 2005), 202–207, http://journal.waocp. org/?sid=Entrez:PubMed&id=pmid:16101334&key=2005.6.2.202.

170. J. Kurata et al., "Esophageal Carcinoma in Indian Jews of Southern Israel: An Epidemiologic Study," *Journal of Clinical Gastroenterology* 12, no. 2, (April 1990), 222–227, https://doi.org/10.1097/00004836-199004000-00025.

171. M. K. Hwang et al., "Cocarcinogenic Effect of Capsaicin Involves Activation of EGFR Signaling but Not TRPV1," *Cancer Research* 70, no. 17, (September 2010), 6859–6869, https://doi.org/10.1158/0008-5472.CAN-09-4393.

172. B. Toth and P. Gannett, "Carcinogenicity of Lifelong Administration of Capsaicin of Hot Pepper in Mice," *In Vivo* 6, no, 1, (January–February 1992), 59–63, https://www.ncbi .nlm.nih.gov/pubmed/1627743.

173. Y. J. Surh, "More Than Spice: Capsaicin in Hot Chili Peppers Makes Tumor Cells Commit Suicide," *Journal of the National Cancer Institute* 94, no. 17, (September 4, 2002), 1263–1265, https://doi.org/10.1093/jnci/94.17.1263.

174. M. Garaulet et al., "Timing of Food Intake Predicts Weight Loss Effectiveness," *International Journal of Obesity* 37, no. 4, (January 29, 2013), 604–611, https://doi.org/10.1038 /ijo.2012.229.

175. D. Jakubowicz et al., "High Caloric Intake at Breakfast Vs. Dinner Differentially Influences Weight Loss of Overweight and Obese Women," *Obesity* 21, no. 12, (March 20, 2013), 2504–2512, https://doi.org/10.1002/oby.20460.

176. K. Y. Wolin, K. Carson, and G. A. Colditz, "Obesity and Cancer," *Oncologist* 15, no. 6, (May 27, 2010), 556–565, https://doi.org/10.1634/theoncologist.2009-0285.

177. E. E. Calle and M. J. Thun, "Obesity and Cancer," *Oncogene* 23, no. 38, (August 23, 2004), 6365–6378, https://doi.org/10.1038/sj.onc.1207751.

178. H. R. Farshchi, M. A. Taylor, and I. A. Macdonald, "Beneficial Metabolic Effects of Regular Meal Frequency on Dietary Thermogenesis, Insulin Sensitivity, and Fasting Lipid Profiles in Healthy Obese Women," *American Journal of Clinical Nutrition* 81, no. 1, (January 2005), 16–24, https://doi .org/10.1093/ajcn/81.1.16.

179. Farshchi, Taylor, and Macdonald, "Beneficial Metabolic Effects of Regular Meal Frequency," 16–24.

180. A. T. Hutchison and L. K. Heilbronn, "Metabolic Impacts of Altering Meal Frequency and Timing—Does When We Eat Matter?" *Biochimie* 124, (2015), 187–197, https://doi .org/10.1016/j.biochi.2015.07.025.

181. B. B. Kahn and J. S. Flier, "Obesity and Insulin Resistance," *Journal of Clinical Investigation* 106, no. 4, (August 15, 2000), 473, https://doi.org/10.1172/JCI10842.

182. H. Kahleova et al., "Eating Two Larger Meals a Day (Breakfast and Lunch) Is More Effective Than Six Smaller Meals in a Reduced-Energy Regimen for Patients With Type 2 Diabetes: A Randomised Crossover Study," *Diabetologia* 57, no. 8, (August 2014), 1552–1560, https://doi.org/10.1007/s00125-014-3253-5.

183. R. A. DeFronzo and E. Ferrannini, "Insulin Resistance: A Multifaceted Syndrome Responsible for NIDDM, Obesity, Hypertension, Dyslipidemia, and Atherosclerotic Cardiovascular Disease," *Diabetes Care* 14, no. 3, (March 1991), 173–194, https://doi.org/10.2337/diacare.14.3.173.

184. DeFronzo and Ferrannini, "Insulin Resistance," 173–194.

185. B. Martin, M. P. Mattson, and S. Maudsley, "Caloric Restriction and Intermittent Fasting: Two Potential Diets for Successful Brain Aging," *Ageing Research Reviews* 5, no. 3, (August 2006), 332–353, https://doi.org/10.1016/j.arr.2006.04.002.

186. M. P. Mattson and R. Wan, "Beneficial Effects of Intermittent Fasting and Caloric Restriction on the Cardiovascular and Cerebrovascular Systems," *Journal of Nutritional Biochemistry* 16, no. 3, (March 2005), 129–137, https://doi.org/10.1016/j.jnutbio.2004.12.007.

187. Mattson and Wan, "Beneficial Effects of Intermittent Fasting and Caloric Restriction," 129–137.

188. S. R. Colberg et al., "Postprandial Walking Is Better for Lowering the Glycemic Effect of Dinner Than Pre-Dinner

Exercise in Type 2 Diabetic Individuals," *Journal of the American Medical Directors Association* 10, no. 6, (July 2009), 394–397, https://doi.org/10.1016/j.jamda.2009.03.015.

189. A. Franke et al., "Postprandial Walking but Not Consumption of Alcoholic Digestifs or Espresso Accelerates Gastric Emptying in Healthy Volunteers," *Journal of Gastrointestinal and Liver Diseases* 17, no. 1, (March 2008), 27, http://www.jgld.ro/2008/1/4.html.

190. C. A. Pellegrini, "Delayed Gastric Emptying in Patients With Abnormal Gastroesophageal Reflux," *Annals of Surgery* 234, no. 2, (August 2001), 147, https://www.ncbi.nlm.nih.gov/pmc/articles/PMC1422000/.

191. A. Park, (May 26, 2010). "How Exercise Works at the Cellular Level." Retrieved from http://healthland.time.com/2010/05/26/how-exercise-works-at-the-cellular-level/.

192. H. Godman, "Regular Exercise Changes the Brain to Improve Memory, Thinking Skills," *Harvard Health Blog*, April 9, 2014, http://www.health.harvard.edu/blog/regular-exercise-changes-brain-improve-memory-thinking-skills-201404097110.

193. K. Y. Wolin et al., "Physical Activity and Colon Cancer Prevention: A Meta-Analysis," *British Journal of Cancer* 100, no. 4, (February 24, 2009), 611–616, https://doi.org/10.1038/sj.bjc.6604917.

194. A. A. Ogunleye and M. D. Holmes, "Physical Activity and Breast Cancer Survival," *Breast Cancer Research* 11, no. 5, (2009), 106, https://doi.org/10.1186/bcr2351.

195. V. B. Sheppard et al., "Physical Activity Reduces Breast Cancer Risk in African American Women," *Ethnicity and Disease* 21, no. 4, (Autumn 2011), 406–411, https://www.ncbi.nlm.nih.gov/pmc/articles/PMC3760197/.

196. D. C. Torti and G. O. Matheson, "Exercise and Prostate Cancer," *Sports Medicine* 34, no. 6, (May 2004), 363–369, https://doi.org/10.2165/00007256-200434060-00003.

197. Ogunleye and Holmes, "Physical Activity and Breast Cancer Survival."

198. S. E. Bonn et al., "Physical Activity and Survival Among Men Diagnosed With Prostate Cancer," *Cancer Epidemiology Biomarkers and Prevention* 24, no. 1, (January 2015), 57–64, https://doi.org/10.1158/1055-9965.EPI-14-0707.

199. "The Water in You," Water Science School, US Geological Survey, Accessed September 15, 2019, http://water.usgs.gov/edu/propertyyou.html.

200. G. J. Tortora and B. Derrickson, *Principles of Anatomy and Physiology*, 13th ed., (Hoboken, New Jersey: John Wiley and Sons, Inc (2012).

201. Tortora and Derrickson, *Principles of Anatomy and Physiology*.

202. B. M. Popkin, K. E. D'Anci, and I. H. Rosenberg, "Water, Hydration and Health," *Nutrition Reviews* 68, no. 8, (August 1, 2010), 439–458, https://doi.org/10.1111/j.1753-4887.2010.00304.x.

203. D. S. Michaud et al., "Fluid Intake and the Risk of Bladder Cancer in Men," *New England Journal of Medicine* 340, no. 18, (May 6, 1999) 1390–1397, https://doi.org/10.1056/NEJM199905063401803.

204. J. Shannon et al., "Relationship of Food Groups and Water Intake to Colon Cancer Risk," *Cancer Epidemiology, Biomarkers and Prevention* 5, no. 7, (July 1996), 496–502, http://cebp.aacrjournals.org/content/5/7/495.full.pdf+html.

205. "Water Use in Hydrotherapy Tanks," Hydrotherapy, Other Uses and Types of Water, Centers for Disease Control and Prevention, October 11, 2016, http://www.cdc.gov/healthywater/other/medical/hydrotherapy.html.

206. "Hyperthermia to Treat Cancer," Treatment Types, Treatments and Side Effects, Treatment and Support, American Cancer Society, May 3, 2016, http://www.cancer.org/treatment/treatmentsandsideeffects/treatmenttypes/hyperthermia.

207. H. D. Suit and M. Shwayder, "Hyperthermia: Potential as an Anti-Tumor Agent," *Cancer* 34, 1, (July 1974), 122–129, https://doi.org/10.1002/1097-0142(197407)34:1<122::AID-CNCR2820340118>3.0.CO;2-R.

208. D. S. Grimes, E. Hindle, and T. Dyer, "Sunlight, Cholesterol and Coronary Heart Disease," *QJM* 89, no. 8, (August 1996), 579–589, https://www.ncbi.nlm.nih.gov/pubmed/8935479.

209. A. L. Ponsonby, R. Lucas, and I. V. D. Mei, "UVR, Vitamin D and Three Autoimmune Diseases—Multiple Sclerosis, Type 1 Diabetes, Rheumatoid Arthritis," *Photochemistry and Photobiology* 81, no. 6, 1267–1275, (April 30, 2007), https://doi.org/10.1562/2005-02-15-IR-441.

210. S. N. Young, "How to Increase Serotonin in the Human Brain Without Drugs," *Journal of Psychiatry and Neuroscience:* 32 no. 6, (November 2007), 394–399, https://www.ncbi.nlm.nih.gov/pmc/articles/PMC2077351/.

211. M. N. Mead, "Benefits of Sunlight: A Bright Spot for Human Health," *Environmental Health Perspectives* 116, no. 4, (April 1, 2008), A160, https://doi.org/10.1289/ehp.116-a160.

212. M. F. Holick, "Sunlight and Vitamin D for Bone Health and Prevention of Autoimmune Diseases, Cancers, and Cardiovascular Disease," *American Journal of Clinical Nutrition* 80, no. 6, (December 2004), 1678S–1688S, https://doi.org/10.1093/ajcn/80.6.1678S.

213. Holick, "Sunlight and Vitamin D" 1678S–1688S.

214. "Why Should You Be Concerned About Air Pollution?" United States Environmental Protection Agency, accessed January 25, 2016, http://www3.epa.gov/airquality/peg_caa/concern.html.

215. "7 Million Premature Deaths Annually Linked to Air Pollution," Media Centre, World Health Organization, March 25, 2014, http://www.who.int/mediacentre/news/releases/2014/air-pollution/en/.

216. B. J. Park et al., "The Physiological Effects of *Shinrin-yoku* (Taking In the Forest Atmosphere or Forest Bathing):

Evidence From Field Experiments in 24 Forests Across Japan," *Environmental Health and Preventive Medicine* 15 no. 1, (January 2010), 18–26, https://doi.org/10.1007/s12199-009-0086-9.

217. Q. Li et al., "A Forest Bathing Trip Increases Human Natural Killer Activity and Expression of Anti-Cancer Proteins in Female Subjects," *Journal of Biological Regulators and Hemeostatic Agents* 22, no. 1, (January–March 2008), 45–55, https://www.ncbi.nlm.nih.gov/pubmed/18394317; Q. Li et al., "Visiting a Forest, but Not a City, Increases Human Natural Killer Activity and Expression of Anti-Cancer Proteins," *International Journal of Immunopathology and Pharmacology* 21, no, 1, (January 1, 2008), 117–127, https://doi.org/10.1177/039463200802100113.

218. L. Xie et al., "Sleep Drives Metabolite Clearance From the Adult Brain," *Science* 342, no. 6156, (October 18, 2013), 373–377, https://doi.org/10.1126/science.1241224.

219. "Why Is Sleep Important?" Sleep Deprivation and Deficiency, National Heart, Lung, and Blood Institute, accessed September 15, 2019, http://www.nhlbi.nih.gov/health/health-topics/topics/sdd/why.

220. National Heart, Lung, and Blood Institute, "Why Is Sleep Important?"

221. B. Sivertsen et al., "Sleep and Pain Sensitivity in Adults," *Pain* 156, no. 8, (August 2015), 1433–1439, https://doi.org/10.1097/j.pain.0000000000000131.

222. C. Hublin et al., "Sleep and Mortality: A Population-Based 22-Year Follow-Up Study," *Sleep* 30, no. 10, (October 1, 2007), 1245, https://doi.org/10.1093/sleep/30.10.1245.

223. S. Davis, D. K. Mirick, and R. G. Stevens, "Night Shift Work, Light at Night, and Risk of Breast Cancer," *Journal of the National Cancer Institute* 93, no. 20, (October 2001), 1557–1562, https://doi.org/10.1093/jnci/93.20.1557.

224. M. Conlon, N. Lightfoot, and N. Kreiger, "Rotating Shift Work and Risk of Prostate Cancer," *Epidemiology* 18, no. 1, (January 2007), 182, 183, https://doi.org/10.1097/01.ede.0000249519.33978.31.

225. M.-É. Parent et al., "Night Work and the Risk of Cancer Among Men," *American Journal of Epidemiology* 176, no. 9, (November 2012), 751–759, https://doi.org/10.1093/aje/kws318.

226. A. H. Wu, M. C. Pike, and D. O. Stram, "Meta-Analysis: Dietary Fat Intake, Serum Estrogen Levels, and the Risk of Breast Cancer," *Journal of the National Cancer Institute* 91, no. 6, (March 17, 1999), 529–534, https://doi.org/10.1093/jnci/91.6.529.

227. W. J. Strawbridge et al., "Frequent Attendance at Religious Services and Mortality Over 28 Years," *American Journal of Public Health* 87, no. 6, (June 1997), 957–961, https://doi.org/10.2105/AJPH.87.6.957.

228. F. Bonaguidi et al., "Religiosity Associated With Prolonged Survival in Liver Transplant Recipients," *Liver Transplantation* 16, no. 10, (October 2010), 1158–1163, https://doi.org/10.1002/lt.22122.

229. A. Newberg, "How Do Meditation and Prayer Change our Brains?" Research Questions, Andrew Newberg.com, accessed September 15, 2019, http://www.andrewnewberg.com/research/.

230. Newberg, "How Do Meditation and Prayer Change our Brains?"

231. *The Twelve Steps of Alcoholics Anonymous,* (Alcoholics Anonymous World Services, Inc., 1981), 1, updated August 2016, http://www.aa.org/assets/en_US/smf-121_en.pdf.

232. Proverbs 17:22, CSB.